DATE DUE

Catching Babies

Catching Babies

The Professionalization of
Childbirth, 1870–1920

Charlotte G. Borst

Harvard University Press
Cambridge, Massachusetts
London, England
1995

Library of Congress Cataloging-in-Publication Data
Borst, Charlotte G.
Catching babies : the professionalization of childbirth, 1870–1920
/ Charlotte G. Borst.
p.   cm.
Includes bibliographical references and index.
ISBN 0-674-10262-2
1. Childbirth—Wisconsin—History—19th century.   2. Childbirth—
Wisconsin—History—20th century.   3. Midwives—Wisconsin—History.
4. Obstetrics—Wisconsin—History.   5. Professions—Sociological aspects.
I. Title.
RG652.B65   1995
618.2′009775—dc20
95-5261

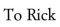

To Rick

Contents

Acknowledgments

Most authors of books such as this acknowledge many people and many institutions for their contributions. I am no exception. The librarians and archivists at several institutions were helpful in providing research tools, money, and space.

The Wisconsin State Historical Society is nationally renowned for its collection of documents and manuscripts in American history, but it was the staff who made it possible for me to fully utilize these treasures. The personnel in the Archives Division helped me locate important manuscripts and documents, and they often went out of their way to find other materials that helped to illuminate my discoveries. Michael Edmunds, in his capacity at the Archives Division and later at Circulation, was enormously helpful. Geraldine Strey at the reference desk traced down obscure references and located useful maps. Lorraine Adkin and John Peters of the government documents section unearthed many valuable federal and state documents. Lori Cook in the microforms section located references even if I had obscure or incomplete citations. I also thank the Historical Society for providing me with a space to do my dissertation research.

The Middleton Health Sciences Library of the University of Wisconsin also has a remarkable collection of journals, texts, and other sources in the history of medicine. I thank the staff at the reference desk for their services in locating many sources. Dorothy Whitcomb, now retired as the Historical Librarian, was particularly helpful in locating many obscure nineteenth-century medical sources when I needed them, often on short notice. Jim Liebig, the archivist for the

University's Medical School and University Extension Archives, located at Steenbock Library, was a personable and helpful source of information about the history and myriad functions of the University of Wisconsin's Extension Service.

Many librarians at the University of Alabama at Birmingham also assisted. Bonnie Ledbetter, the social science reference librarian at Sterne Library, went out of her way to be helpful. The staff of the Lister Hill Medical Library located obscure historical medical journals and books.

I spent over nine months gathering data from Wisconsin's vital statistics records. The busy staff at the Vital Records Office of the Wisconsin Department of Health and Human Services in Madison put up with a historian in their midst and found me a space to work in. I am particularly grateful to them.

Judith Walzer Leavitt has been a true mentor. In working with her, I have learned how to be both a teacher and a scholar. She helped guide this project from its inception and provided needed advice and encouragement. Her comments were enormously helpful in revising and shaping my ideas and my writing.

Many friends and colleagues helped me complete this project by reading drafts of chapters, listening to my ideas, and providing a shoulder to lean on when I needed one. Elizabeth T. Black read or listened to many chapters of my dissertation. Colleagues at the University of Wisconsin—Milwaukee, particularly Carol Shammas, gave support and technical assistance with some of the issues raised in Chapters 3 and 4. My colleagues at the University of Alabama at Birmingham, particularly Carolyn Conley and the members of the Alabama History of Medicine and Science Group, read chapters of this manuscript and offered important critiques when they were needed. Rachel Hawks Chenot and Diane Robinson Dunn were extremely helpful and thorough research assistants. Throughout the many years involved in this project, Kathleen W. Jones, now at Virginia Polytechnic and State University, offered friendship and more help than I can ever adequately acknowledge.

Without grants and aid, this project would never have been completed. Thanks to the Wisconsin Historical Society for awarding me the Alice E. Smith Award. The Maurice Richardson Fund at the University of Wisconsin was particularly generous in providing a year of fellowship assistance, as well as money for keypunching the large birth certificate data set. A faculty research grant from the University of Alabama at Birmingham provided the means to complete my research, and a grant from the National Library of Medicine (National Institutes of Health Publication Grant Program, number LM05491) provided the necessary time to complete the writing. Under the provisions of this grant, I acknowledge that the contents of this book do not necessarily represent the official views of the National Library of Medicine.

The biggest debt I owe is to my family. My father, Charles Van Slyke Borst, fostered my early interest in books, particularly in American history. I wish that he had lived to see his encouragement come to fruition. Helen Kasabuski, my husband's grandmother, emigrated from Poland as a young girl. I am particularly grateful that her financial assistance enabled me to purchase the personal computer and the software that made my statistical analysis possible. I was always mindful of her quiet dignity as I wrote about the lives of immigrant women like her. My children, Stefan and Zosia, provided needed interruptions and a welcome relief from academic pursuits. In addition, their births, one with the help of a nurse-midwife and the other by emergency cesarean section, gave me a unique perspective on many issues in the history of childbirth. Most of all, I wish to thank my husband, Richard P. Censullo. He has been my best friend and my most loyal supporter as well as an exemplary husband. He has consistently supported this project, acting at different times as research assistant, editor, and primary parent so that I could work without worry. I dedicate this work to him.

Catching Babies

Midwives, Physicians, and Professionalism

From the colonial period to the Great Depression, midwives delivered a large proportion of America's babies. As late as 1900, half of all the children born in a given year in the United States were delivered with the help of a midwife attendant. Yet, by 1930, midwife-attended births had dropped to less than 15 percent of all births in the United States, and most of these were in the south.[1] Physicians and, increasingly after 1950, obstetrician-specialist physicians attended most parturient women. Midwifery was left to become a curious historical artifact with a sometimes dubious reputation.[2]

The shift in childbirth attendants in these years is one of the striking examples of the relationship of gender, class, and culture in the early twentieth-century movement in the United States towards professionalization and the strengthening of professional authority. Childbirth had always been a potentially dangerous as well as joyous occasion, and parturient women sought help in minimizing this danger.[3] Though physicians were increasingly called upon in the nineteenth century to provide a measure of safety, many women could see little difference between a physician and a knowledgeable midwife. But by the end of the nineteenth century, many Americans' attitudes about expertise, especially as practiced by scientists, were transformed. Americans of the Progressive Era came to view scientific and other specialized knowledge as the province of professionals, and the birthing room became an arena for demonstrating the goals of the new scientific professional.[4]

But the replacement of midwives by physicians in America's

birthing rooms in the early twentieth century involved more than the elevation of the science and art of medicine.[5] The explanation for the change to physician-assisted childbirth in the United States in the early twentieth century lies in large part with the specific gender, class, and cultural components involved in the process of professionalization in this period. Childbirth was one important place where traditional female knowledge, practice, and sphere of influence directly confronted the goals of the new professional. The outcome of this conflict helped to define the gender, ethnic, and class characteristics that identified the professional birth attendant and even the nature of the professional's work.

Sociologists and historians have identified a number of criteria to judge the movement of an occupation toward professionalization. These include the standardization of training, the creation of a distinct and exclusive body of knowledge, the control over the production of both knowledge and its producers, and most important, autonomy—the freedom to resolve the tension between the technical and the indeterminant aspects of work.[6] Additionally, professionals can be defined as full-time specialists, who work full-time because their work is their source of income.[7] Studying the change in childbirth attendants in the late nineteenth and early twentieth centuries is a particularly useful way to examine the process of professionalization. As Magali Larson and others have pointed out, these seemingly objective criteria were also based in a historical context where the men involved were "carriers of social structure." In particular, the middle class, which emerged as a result of industrial capitalism, was favorably situated to develop the tools and the power for the professions.[8]

But while issues of class were certainly important in the development of the American medical profession, issues of gender and culture have received much less attention, yet they are crucial for understanding childbearing families' willingness to accept professional birth attendants in the early twentieth century. Midwives were, after all, women, and many of them by 1900 were immigrant or black women, as were many of their patients.[9] Communities where midwives and their patients lived were closely knit; families relied on one another for many services. Women played a central role in providing these services, particularly in matters involving health. Given the central place of childbirth as a cultural event, economic and class issues alone

2

do not explain why women in these communities were willing to accept (mostly) male physicians as their birth attendants.[10]

In this book, I offer a critique of the model of professionalization used by historians and sociologists by analyzing the work of a group of midwives and physicians who practiced in four Wisconsin counties between 1870 and 1920. Midwifery, an occupation structured by traditional gender and cultural definitions, did not professionalize. Medicine, on the other hand, was the epitome of a profession usually practiced by men. While the gender difference between midwives and most physicians is not the only factor in understanding why birth attendants changed, the influence of gender on each type of birth attendant's occupation was an integral part of the professionalizing process. The interaction between culture and professionalization was more complex. The relationship between physicians and their patients was an intricate one, based on the bonds of class and ethnicity, just as it had been for midwives and their patients. Thus, when the medical profession began to fracture into specialties in the early twentieth century, concepts of culture and class played important roles in determining the qualities of a professional obstetrical specialist.[11]

This study of midwife and physician birth attendants is structured to reflect both the chronological as well as the theoretical changes in the professionalization of childbirth. Chapters 1 through 4 are devoted to the analysis of midwife education, family lives, and practice in rural and urban Wisconsin. Chapters 5 through 7 examine the role of education in promoting physicians as expert birth attendants, and the practice of obstetrics by general practitioners and specialists.

Sociologists and historians often use the level of education among practitioners as an important criterion in determining a level of professional success for a given occupation.[12] By the end of the nineteenth century among northern, white midwives, this female occupation was moving in the classical way from informal to formal training. Indeed, by 1900, many of the midwives practicing in rural Wisconsin were trained at a school. But though the majority of midwives were receiving a more rationalized education, midwives never controlled their schools, nor did they help to establish the credentials for practice. Even nursing, which historians have described as lacking professionalism because of the nature of its work, had the autonomy to run its own training schools and to set its own standards of practice.[13] Midwives, however, relied on physicians to make decisions about their occupation. This reliance on leadership from outside the occupation reflected its practitioners' lack of real autonomy and its roots in a traditional culture that valued personal relationships for establishing fitness to perform a task.

Professionals, however, are defined by more than their educational qualifications. Midwives' work, like the work that nurses performed, was inherently defined as women's work. Up to the end of the nineteenth century, in fact, the qualifications for the two jobs were quite similar—maturity, marriage, and experience with housework. But as Susan Reverby, Barbara Melosh, and others have shown, under the leadership of middle-class, native-born women, the image of nursing changed in the late nineteenth century, and nursing came to be associated with work performed by young, unmarried, and predominantly middle-class women.[14] However, despite the fact that midwives were also receiving school training, the images of midwives in this period remained linked to those at the bottom of America's social scale—immigrants and African-Americans. The historical constructs of gender that others have found inhibiting the growth of female-dominated occupations like nursing were magnified for midwives by their ties to husbands and children and the place of women in traditional cultures. These ethnic, working-class women stood no chance of becoming part of a professional process that was, in part, an attempt to claim authority and power.[15]

But to portray midwives only as victims is to lose sight of how they saw their work. Whatever their training or even their level of practice, midwives as a group shared common ground as middle-aged, married women with families of their own. Though stereotypical descriptions of these practitioners held that they were old women who sometimes were incapable of doing any other work, I found that most Wisconsin midwives were middle-aged mothers who practiced when they still had young children at home. Immigrant women dominated the practice of midwifery in this state, much as African-American midwives were in the majority in the south. But for immigrant or African-American women, midwifery was practiced out of the home, as one of women's many traditional domestic skills.

The patterns of midwifery practice in rural and urban Wisconsin suggest that it is unlikely that female birth attendants ever sought a professional status for their work. Indeed, midwifery practice in rural Wisconsin resembled more closely the patterns of gender-specific mutual aid that farm women provided for one another than it did an organized, income-producing activity. Most rural midwives were neighbor women who attended only a handful of cases, "catching" the babies of their nearby relatives and neighbors. Even trained rural midwives did not have large practices. Though they would expect to receive payment for their work, even the most active rural midwives attended no more than one or two cases per month. Furthermore, like neighbor-woman midwives, active midwives restricted their practice to their village or nearby farms. Most importantly, regardless of their level of activity or training, rural midwives practiced among the women of their own ethnic group or their American-born daughters.

While the process of urbanization in late nineteenth-century America has been linked to the emergence of many professional groups, it did not have the same impact on midwifery. Though urban areas like Milwaukee offered the potential for building much larger midwifery practices than those in Wisconsin's rural areas, only a few urban midwives attended large numbers of births. Furthermore, even the most active midwives in the city continued to base their practice in neighborhoods defined by close ethnic and geographic ties. Like the small shopkeepers who relied on fellow countrypeople for business, these busy midwives advertised and worked within the confines of an ethnic community, and their clients came from down the street or around the corner. Moreover, unlike physicians or even nurses, they never formed practitioner societies that might advance their cause as professionals. Thus, though a few of these female birth attendants earned substantial amounts of money from their midwifery skills, it is more likely that they viewed their practice in entrepreneurial, rather than professional, terms.

In the absence of a professionalizing strategy for midwifery, the professional strategy of physicians went unchallenged. Between 1870 and 1930, medicine struggled to achieve cultural authority, and childbirth had become an arena for demonstrating the goals of the new scientific professional. Though "catching a baby," as midwives and some doctors termed it,[16] often involved waiting around for nature to do its work, physicians and some parturient women came to believe that science and scientific medicine could offer a safer or more secure outcome.[17] By 1930, physicians virtually monopolized childbirth among white families in the United States.

The transformation of medical education played an important role in strengthening the professional status and consolidating the professional authority of all physicians. Changes first in the basic science curriculum and then in the clinical curriculum linked medical training to new developments in laboratory science. This new science also invested physicians with increased authority in the birthing room that enabled them to claim obstetrical work for themselves.[18]

While much is known about the opinions of national medical leaders and the deficiencies of the curricula of late nineteenth-century medical schools, almost no work has examined both the education of a specific group of practicing physicians and the possible effects of educational reform on obstetrical practice.[19] This study of Wisconsin physicians assesses the level of training and education among practicing physicians and then examines how this training affected the practice of obstetrics. It shows that though the public in the Progressive Era perceived doctors as representatives of the new and legitimately complex scientific community, a significant gap existed between the perceptions of scientific expertise and the reality.[20] In fact, not until 1920 could young Wisconsin physicians claim to have seen as many as twenty births in the course of their bedside training, a number that was less than or equal to that of some of the school-trained midwives in the state.[21]

Though their training was not demonstrably more "scientific" than that of midwives, Wisconsin physicians began to replace these female birth attendants in increasing numbers after the turn of the twentieth century. But the professional status of the male physicians who were called in to attend maternity cases rested more with their standing within the community than with concepts of scientific efficacy that were only vaguely understood. Indeed, many of the first physicians to attend maternity cases were rural physicians, who practiced in places that never built institutions, such as hospitals or medical schools, that would come to define the essence of scientific, laboratory medicine in the twentieth century.[22] Thus, the contours of rural general practice were very similar to those of midwives: all physicians practiced within a limited geographical area, and many doctors shared the same ethnic background as their patients. Consequently, the acceptance of the

physician birth attendant incorporated a professional ideal represented by familiar, powerful, male figures who could be trusted to
translate and interpret the new science into acceptable terms for the
community.

By the early twentieth century, however, even general practitioners
found themselves under attack for their lack of skill and knowledge
about obstetrics. Some nationally prominent physicians, such as Joseph B. DeLee in Chicago and John Whitridge Williams at the Johns
Hopkins Medical School, called for scientifically oriented obstetrical
specialists to replace midwives and even general practitioners, whom
they lambasted almost as often as they excoriated midwives. But in
the early twentieth century the concept of a medical specialist was in
flux and the first group of obstetrical specialists to emerge in urban
Wisconsin based its criteria for professionalism on the traditional concept of experience with large numbers of patients. Indeed, this group,
based in the ethnic communities of Milwaukee, had been responsible
for the change from midwife- to physician-assisted childbirth in these
communities. By the second decade of the twentieth century, however, another physician group—the institutional specialists—laid
claim to the mantle of professionalism. Just as gender and culture had
played a role in causing the general practitioner to be seen as more
professional than the midwife, gender, culture, and class helped shape
a model of the obstetrical specialist. Though many of the new institutional specialists actually attended far fewer births per month than
the doctors in the immigrant communities, their elite social status
helped them gain access and assume power in the hospitals and medical schools that came to dominate twentieth-century ideals of "scientific" medical practice.[23]

In order to study both midwives and physicians within the context
of their community, I focus on four representative counties in Wisconsin.[24] The changes chronicled in these specific communities can
be used to understand the broader transformation in Americans' ideas
about experts in the early twentieth century. I chose Wisconsin because it was a representative northern state with a large number of
practicing midwives around 1900. The state is known for its Progressive tradition, and its good record keeping provided excellent and
available sources of information. Unlike Massachusetts, which banned
midwifery in the 1890s, thus forcing it underground, or many

southern states, which left midwifery completely unregulated, Wisconsin regulated, but did not ban, midwifery in the years before 1930.[25] Thus, midwives practiced openly in Wisconsin, and there were records of their education and their practice. In addition to good data about midwives, Wisconsin had fairly typical medical licensing laws. The state was neither a notorious center for irregular and uneducated doctors, nor was it an elite center for academic medicine. Wisconsin physicians thus represented a fairly typical cross-section of late nineteenth- and early twentieth-century practitioners.[26]

To study a large group of practitioners and to examine trends over a significant amount of time, I use the methodology of social science history, particularly statistical analysis and historical demography. Though I also used many of the more traditional literary sources common to historical research, much of my primary evidence comes from birth certificates, midwife and physician licenses, city directories, and federal and state census manuscript schedules. In all, six discrete data sets were gathered and coded for numerical analysis. (For details of these sets, see the appendix.)

By analyzing the actual practice of midwifery and physician obstetrics within the context of a particular community, *Catching Babies* is part of many historiographic currents, including the history of childbirth, medical, women's, and even immigrant history. Previous work on midwives and physicians has concentrated almost solely on the more narrow problem of the relationship between midwives and physicians. Some of the previous scholarship grew out of a critique of medical authority in general, but most of the work on this topic developed from the enormous surge of interest in women's history in the early 1970s. Concentrating on the physician debates about midwives at the turn of the twentieth century, scholars attempted to fashion a more positive historical image of these often maligned female birth attendants. They found, for example, that midwives frequently had better outcomes in terms of maternal or infant mortality than physicians and that many midwives were highly esteemed by women within their communities.[27]

Though these earlier studies identified the debate about midwives among medical practitioners at the turn of the twentieth century, there were at least four general areas where their approach was limited. By concentrating on the legal status of midwives and the struggles of physicians to regulate midwifery, many of these studies devoted little attention to the training for or the actual practice of midwifery.[28] Also, in looking at midwives through the eyes of physicians, some scholars portrayed these women only as victims of an all-powerful and sometimes sexist medical establishment. One result was that midwives were usually portrayed as poor, isolated practitioners who did not have the resources to stand up to their critics.[29] In addition, a focus on national medical leaders tended to blur the important cultural distinctions inherent in midwifery practice. While historical studies tended to concentrate on midwives in the urban northeast United States, midwives practiced in many other parts of the country, under substantially different circumstances from those faced by northeast practitioners.[30] The fourth, and most serious, limitation, was the failure to link the physician debate directly to the decline of midwifery. Though a number of authors identified important issues, they did not posit a causal relationship between the physicians' debate, the professionalization of obstetrics, and the disappearance of midwives.

While the history of the decline of midwives has received almost universally sympathetic treatment, the rise of physicians as birth attendants often has been represented in a much less favorable light. Some polemical histories of this subject depict physicians at the turn of the twentieth century as scheming sexists, conniving to push midwives out of their rightful place at birthing women's bedsides.[31] Less partisan analyses concentrate only on the arguments of national medical leaders, who saw midwives as interfering with their efforts to reform obstetrics into a professionalized medical specialty.[32] But very little work has examined the training and the practice of obstetrics by the average general practitioner in the early twentieth century.

This study, by concentrating on one area in the midwest, looks at midwife and physician obstetrical practice within its cultural context, and builds on recent scholarship that has introduced a new methodology for childbirth history. By refocusing the relationship between childbearing women and their birth attendants, these recent studies not only helped to correct the tarnished image of the physician but, more important, also showed the complex relationship between women and their birth attendants. For example, Judith Walzer

9

Leavitt's use of women's diaries and letters together with physicians' journals and casebooks demonstrated that nineteenth- and early twentieth-century women invited physicians into their birthing rooms, and both women and their doctors negotiated about appropriate techniques and interventions. In Leavitt's view, women made conscious choices for themselves and their babies, based on their fears about death and debility.[33] Laurel Ulrich's analysis of the diary of Martha Ballard, a late eighteenth-century midwife, showed that midwifery was part of "a larger neighborhood economy, . . . the most visible feature of a comprehensive and little-known system of early health care, . . . a mechanism of social control, a strategy for family support, and a deeply personal calling."[34] But we see this larger neighborhood economy because Mrs. Ballard's diary was a source generated by a midwife herself, not by doctors critical of midwives. Thus, through the viewpoint of a midwife's own diary, we are able for the first time to gain some perspective on what midwives in the past thought about their work. In a similar way, my study of childbirth attendants in Wisconsin in the late nineteenth and early twentieth centuries analyzes sources generated by midwives and doctors to explore the rise of professionalism within the context of particular communities.

Though childbirth has generally been recognized as a culturally laden family and community event, *Catching Babies* is the first study to examine the move to physician-attended birth within the context of a particular community. Historians since the early 1970s have found community studies a useful way to analyze many of the complex problems of social history. Community studies, whether case studies of particular phenomena like mobility or reconstructions of the social and spatial structures of large cities, describe the social relationships between groups of people and specifically address the interrelationships among class, gender, ethnicity, family, and environment.[35]

The relationship between a birth attendant's professional status and his or her ethnic background is one of the recurring themes of this book, and it forms an important analytical tool. As shown by Kathleen Conzen's work on Milwaukee, Olivier Zunz's study of Detroit, and other books analyzing immigrant families and their communities in the United States, mid- and late nineteenth-century cities were highly segregated by ethnic groups.[36] Each ethnic neighborhood, however, was occupationally heterogeneous, with poor and middle-income immigrants living side by side. Some of the larger immigrant enclaves had groups of professionals, including physicians. This heterogeneous class structure, Zunz argues, allowed for upward mobility within one's own ethnic group and often reinforced ethnic divisions.[37]

Wisconsin's well-defined rural and urban ethnic communities provided a number of places to study the parameters of the professionalization of childbirth. They also provided a mechanism to analyze the process of professionalization as a part of the Progressive movement.[38] Some historians have argued that these experts were part of an elite class that came from the outside to impose values and ideas on traditional communities.[39] Previous histories of the shift from midwife to physician-assisted childbirth also often have used the notion of outside social control to explain historical change in America's immigrant communities. But my examination of the historical and social contexts of those involved in the change in childbirth attendants in Wisconsin found few outsiders who were seeking to impose their ideas about change. Midwives in Wisconsin were not pushed out of practice by elitist or misogynist obstetricians. Instead, their traditional, artisanal skills ceased to be valued by a society that had come to embrace the model of disinterested, professionalized science. In addition, the physicians who disseminated this new science did not impose values foreign to the community. Instead, the community that had previously hired midwives turned to physicians whose ethnic and cultural values were very similar to those of the midwives they replaced.

But just as issues relating to gender prevented midwives from establishing their craft as a profession in the early twentieth century, cultural assumptions guided the development of medical specialties like obstetrics. By the middle of the twentieth century, most births in the United States were handled by physicians practicing in hospitals. For physicians who wished to practice obstetrics, new obstetrical standards superseded those that had granted community physicians professional authority in the early twentieth century. Mere interest in the subject, or even an extensive practice within the neighborhood, would not define a medical specialty. With professional status increasingly based on new institutional structures within medicine, physicians turned away from patients and to their peers for approbation. But the social upheavals of the late 1950s and 1960s, together with a growing awareness by the 1980s and 1990s of the high cost of specialized medical practice, demonstrated that the relationship of professionalism to issues of gender, class, and culture would need to be reconsidered.

CHAPTER ONE

Training Midwives

On February 1, 1895, twenty-five-year-old Bertha Wichtel of Milwaukee, Wisconsin, began midwifery school at the Milwaukee College of Midwifery. During her five months of study at this small proprietary school, Wichtel attended lectures on the physiology and the anatomy of reproduction and assisted at thirty deliveries in the school's lying-in division.[1]

While Bertha Wichtel was obtaining her midwifery skills at school, Dora Larson, living in the small, rural village of Woodford, Wisconsin, became a midwife in a more traditional way. Thirty-seven years old and the mother of eight children, Larson learned midwifery techniques from assisting her midwife mother, by helping local physicians attending confinement cases, and from her own experiences giving birth.[2]

The training and midwife practices of Dora Larson and Bertha Wichtel were representative of the circumstances of many late nineteenth and early twentieth-century American midwives. Their education in particular illustrated midwifery's traditional roots as a woman's neighborly occupation and its evolution at the end of the nineteenth century into a rationalized and potentially medicalized discipline. Like their physician and nursing counterparts, trained midwives, educated in schools, were beginning to replace untrained and apprentice-trained practitioners. An analysis of the training of Wisconsin's midwives, however, shows that the question for midwifery was whether education could ultimately transform this traditional woman's craft into a recognized profession.

In the late nineteenth and early twentieth centuries, medicine, nursing, and midwifery all faced the question of determining what kinds of training their practitioners needed. But the issues of training had repercussions beyond pedagogy. By the early twentieth century, the adoption of formal education had the potential to move an occupation towards professional status, a move that conferred increased cultural authority. For medical and nursing leaders, professional status was a well-articulated result of educational reform. Disciplined, school-trained practitioners, they argued, understood the precepts of the new science, and these practitioners deserved and could even demand the layperson's respect of the "expert."[3] But what happened to midwifery?

As in medicine and nursing, the question for midwifery in the early twentieth century was whether advances in training would help it to achieve a professional status similar to that enjoyed by the other health professions.[4] In the end, however, school training for midwives did not lead to professionalization. Instead, midwives became more subservient to physicians and their autonomy decreased. Indeed, by the middle of the twentieth century, midwifery as an occupation had virtually died out in the United States.

To understand the impact of midwifery education, we must pose the same questions about midwives that medical historians have about physicians and nurses: How did midwife training move from casual learning to apprenticeships to school training? How did this transformation of training affect the occupation? Were trained midwives able to claim an exclusive body of knowledge? Were these practitioners then able to control their own institutions and determine who could practice midwifery? How was this attempted transformation affected by the gender, class, and race of the practitioners? Were these changes part of the classic move of an occupation toward professionalization?

By the end of the nineteenth century, there were observable trends in midwife education clearly evident among the northern white midwives of Wisconsin. Licenses filed to comply with a 1909 state statute and the registration data on midwives provided by the Milwaukee Health Department, show that between 1870 and 1920 three types of midwives practiced in the state. Defined by the sources of their training, these practitioners were: neighbor-woman midwives, usually native-born women who learned their techniques from giving birth themselves and from assisting at the deliveries of relatives and a few close friends; apprentice-trained midwives, typically native-born, who learned their craft from other, older midwives or from physicians; and school-educated midwives, overwhelmingly first- or second-generation immigrants, instructed in formal settings with both didactic and practical work. Although each kind of midwife could be found practicing in Wisconsin during much of the fifty-year period, among the nearly nine hundred women identified, there was a distinct evolution from primarily neighbor-woman to apprentice-trained to school-trained practitioners.

Neighbor-Woman Midwives

Neighbor-woman midwives, who were entirely self-taught, were the most traditional birth attendants in late nineteenth-century Wisconsin.[5] Living in isolated rural areas, helping their family members or neighbors, these women practiced midwifery in a way that would have been familiar in the seventeenth or eighteenth century. Susan Washburn was a good example. Sixty years old, this Millston, Wisconsin, midwife wrote of her education in 1909: "I would state that my [midwifery] Education has been limited; has more in careing [sic] for those that are going to be confined in my own neighborhood. I have followed this about 30 years. with good results my experience has been much in midwifery: I never lost a case."[6]

Washburn's age and her rural locale were typical of the group of neighbor-woman midwives practicing in Wisconsin and elsewhere in the United States.[7] Isolated rural women traditionally had called on each other for help when they were having a baby, and often the experience gained in having and caring for children had to suffice in lieu of more formal knowledge. This was particularly true for southern African-American midwives; one Virginia midwife was the mother of nineteen children, seven of whom had survived.[8]

Susan Washburn was also representative of a type of midwife who was disappearing in America by the late nineteenth century. For neighbor-woman midwives, the boundary between the formal label of "midwife" and the more informal idea of neighborliness was often blurred. Some neighbor women did not even consider themselves truly midwives, for besides their own confinements, they attended only a few other births in their family or among their friends. This hazy distinction between merely helping out one's neighbor and assuming a title conveying authority lasted well into the twentieth century, as illustrated by a 1919 Children's Bureau report. Reviewing maternity care in rural America, the committee noted that "many country women are cared for entirely by neighbors, who may or may not have acquired some skill from experience." They distinguished these cases from those handled by recognized birth attendants by adding that "in some parts of the country, [women are cared for] by midwives."[9] A nurse in the mid-1920s reported a distinction between the helpful neighbor and the formal practitioner that hinged on the issue of payment. She related that kindly friends attended births to help out their needy neighbors, but they vehemently denied being midwives because they did not work for pay.[10]

Susan Washburn, however, did not deny that she practiced midwifery. In fact Washburn, together with 38 other Wisconsin neighbor women, took the step to achieve formal recognition by registering after 1909 for midwife licenses. These 39 female birth attendants shared two other distinguishing characteristics in addition to their completely informal training: their advanced age and their rural locale.

The mean age of the 373 midwives who made up the state register was forty-eight. However, the neighbor-woman midwives were, on average, six years older (fifty-four) than the overall mean, and they were considerably older than the school-trained group, whose mean age was forty-six.[11] The trends among Wisconsin midwives mirrored national trends among white midwives. For example, James Lincoln Huntington's 1912 study of Massachusetts midwives showed similar results. Among the midwives where age and training could be identified, those midwives lacking diplomas were elderly women: of 24 midwives without diplomas where age could be verified, 18 were aged fifty or more, and eight of these women were aged sixty or more.[12]

But unlike the Massachusetts midwives, Wisconsin's neighbor-woman midwives were overwhelmingly rural: only one midwife in this group of 39 lived in Milwaukee, the state's most urban area.[13] This link between neighbor-woman midwives and rural residence was reinforced by an analysis of the 588 women who registered with the

Milwaukee Health Department between 1877 and 1907. Over the thirty-year period of the Milwaukee registry, only 21 women reported no training.[14]

Although it is difficult to assess accurately the expertise of neighbor-woman midwives, their informal training probably left some of them unable to do any more for their patients than they knew from the circumstances of their own children's births. While some of these attendants supplemented their own experiences by reading textbooks, other neighbor-woman midwives developed their skills by the sheer necessity of practice.[15] Trapped by bad roads that were impassable due to mud or snow during many portions of the year, childbearing women in isolated rural settlements often were left to rely totally on nearby neighbors.[16] In these situations, perhaps even the ministrations of an attendant such as Minnie Gray, an Arkansas, Wisconsin, neighbor-woman midwife who said that she looked to her Bible for help, were better than none at all.[17]

Neighbor-woman midwives were the most traditional kind of birth attendant. They acted as midwives to their own family or nearby friends in the absence of a trained attendant, and their knowledge was entirely self-generated. Despite their limitations, however, these women were the most autonomous midwives: the conditions under which they practiced permitted them complete freedom. But by the early twentieth century, even in isolated rural areas, families turned to these practitioners only when they could not find a trained midwife. It is not surprising, therefore, that as frontier areas of Wisconsin became more settled and more accessible, trained midwives replaced neighbor women. By the beginning of the twentieth century, these family-based healers were found only in limited numbers in the most rural parts of the state.

Apprentice-Trained Midwives

Throughout American history, many midwives, like many physicians, received their training by apprenticing themselves to older, more experienced practitioners. Indeed, in the United States until the last decades of the nineteenth century, many physicians and almost all trained midwives learned their trade this way. Anne Nowak, of Lublin (in north-central Wisconsin) reported her training in these familiar terms: "I have not taken up the course in any school but have practiced with a professional midwife until I was fully capable of doing the work alone."[18]

Apprenticeship to an experienced practitioner was common in this period among southern African-American midwives, and their stories about their training reflected themes common to both black and white midwives. A student midwife would accompany an experienced birth attendant on her rounds, learning her skills and gaining the confidence of the local women. As Onnie Lee Logan, a Mobile, Alabama, midwife remembered, "I went around with a midwife who done already got her permit for three deliveries. Apprentice." She learned by watching and helping: "They taught me lil pieces here and there. I was always anxious to learn and get started on whatever it would take to be a good midwife. It just come to me from them."[19] Eventually, the student might even inherit her teacher's patients.

Though the teacher midwife could be a respected older neighbor, it was not uncommon for both African-American and white midwives to learn from their own mothers. Dora Larson, for example, learned midwifery from her mother and, as several historians have found, many African-American birth attendants could trace a midwifery lineage back to grandmothers or even great-grandmothers who had worked as slave midwives.[20]

But as a northern, white midwife, Anne Nowak's education at the side of a preceptor midwife was unusual when compared with the apprenticeships of other Wisconsin midwives. While some nineteenth-century midwives did learn their craft from older, more experienced midwives, many more female birth attendants apprenticed themselves with local physicians. Of the 49 apprentice-trained women who registered with the state, 35 (or 71 percent) reported that their instruction came from physicians. Mary Greeley, a practitioner in western Wisconsin, was typical, declaring that she "[has] been practicing midwifery for 30 years usually under the direction of physicians of River Falls, Wis. and Ellsworth, Wis."[21]

The timing of this kind of instruction in the midwife's career varied. Some women received their initial training from physicians and then went out to deliver babies, as Ellen Stiefvator, a northern Wisconsin practitioner, noted about herself: "Practiced with Dr. Rawls Gadsden Ala 30 yrs ago and have practiced ever since; [the] last 18 years in

Merrill Wis[.]"[22] Her training probably lasted at least two years. Many midwives, however, learned informally from doctors as the need arose in the course of a delivery. Calling in the physician for a problem they could not handle alone, midwives learned new techniques as the physician explained what he was doing. Gabrielle Sedall had learned her skills in this way: "[I] have had no institutional training but have take[n] instructions from doctors who attended in the cases in which . . . [I was] called in as midwife."[23] Indeed, it is probable that Ellen Stiefvator also supplemented her training in this way, as she noted that she had "no course except in practice with doctors."[24] Two other women learned their craft from physician family members. Mary Weidman recounted that she had "studied with my father who was a Doctor," while Mary Gordan reported that her education had come from "practice with my former husband Dr. J. V. Smith."[25]

For midwives who practiced in rural areas, this cooperation between midwives and physicians was neither unusual nor surprising. In the rural south, African-American midwives reported that physicians encouraged them to deliver babies. Indeed, Louvenia Taylor, who practiced in rural southern Alabama, reported that she was "forced" by physicians to become a midwife. Though race was undoubtedly a factor, it appears that in the rural south, as in the rural north, physicians were often too busy to attend to deliveries. Taylor reports that the doctors begged her to get a license and help them out.[26] In rural areas of Wisconsin as well, physicians relied on midwives to take on obstetrical cases. Indeed, a 1919 Children's Bureau survey of childbirth attendants in northern Wisconsin found that in one village, for example, local doctors had ceded all of the obstetrical work to Mrs. M., a local German midwife. The doctors referred their maternity cases willingly, telling the survey authors, "We don't like that kind of work and have always more or less turned it over to [her]."[27]

This close interaction between midwives and doctors was not limited to rural maternity practice. Though historians who have analyzed physician debates over the "midwife question" of the late nineteenth and early twentieth centuries have focused particularly on urban physicians' hostility toward midwives, many Milwaukee physicians trained midwives.[28] While some of these physicians were European-educated émigrés and may have been continuing a traditional association common to their ethnic group, other Milwaukee doctors who worked closely with midwives were graduates of American medical schools. Furthermore, most of these American physicians were well regarded and were not marginal practitioners at the fringes of the Milwaukee medical community.[29] Indeed, the most striking feature of apprentice-trained midwives in Milwaukee was that virtually all of them were trained by physicians.

The apprenticeships offered by these physicians varied widely in length and breadth. Some midwives trained for several months; others spent up to a year preparing for practice. The course work ranged from private lectures to a combination of didactic and practical work. Frances Jahnz, for example, "studied with Dr. F. S. Wasielewski for (2) two months [in 1901], then took up ten (10) practical cases of confinement in his presence according to his instructions."[30] Working with another Milwaukee doctor as well, her entire course of instruction, she stated, lasted one year. Mary Browikowski had "received instructions in the art of midwifery for fully five months from Dr. F. M. Hinz, M.D." in 1892.[31] Dr. Hinz also offered seven months of private instruction to Henriette Wenzel in 1898.[32] Other Milwaukee physicians also offered lecture courses to midwives that ranged in length from six to twelve months.[33]

Though some historians of midwifery in America have emphasized the hostility, or at least the indifference, most doctors held for these female practitioners, an examination of data from Wisconsin and elsewhere indicates that midwives and physicians sometimes worked together in America's birthing rooms. Mary Holub, for example, reported on her education and continuing relationship with her physician mentor: "[I received] practical training under Dr. Andrew Munro. attended confinement cases with him and studied under him. Have certificate from him and recommendation to practice. Attended cases with him for a period of seven years."[34]

Apprentice training, however, was not a major route to the profession for Milwaukee midwives. Overall, of the 588 women who registered with the Milwaukee Health Department between 1877 and 1907, only 51 (8.7 percent) reported an apprentice education. The Health Department data also reveal the declining popularity of apprenticeships, from 15.7 percent of the registrants in the early years to 6.6 percent in the last years of the registry. The state licenses, covering a somewhat later period (1909–1915), also demonstrate the decline in the twentieth century in apprentice training. The mean age of the physician-trained midwives, 53.4, approached that of the neighbor women. Furthermore, by this period few urban midwives were learning their craft from physicians: of 189 Milwaukee midwives who registered with the state, only 12 (6.3 percent) were physician-trained. (See Figure 1.1 for a breakdown of education by urban and rural residence.)

School-Educated Midwives

The language Mary Holub used to describe her seven-year relationship with Dr. Munro reveals what became one of the most significant underlying problems for midwifery education as it moved towards formalized schooling in the early twentieth century. When midwives taught other midwives, women remained in charge of the training process. Indeed, the pupil midwife in this relationship might herself expect someday to train other midwives. However, as physicians as-

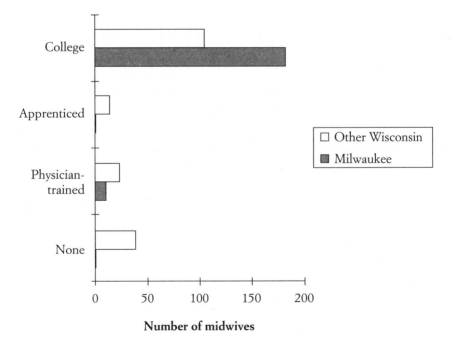

Figure 1.1 Midwife training by type and region, 1909–1915

sumed the role of teaching midwives, they retained the ultimate control over both the education and the conditions of practice for midwifery. Even if midwives helped to start or to capitalize midwifery schools, interested physicians were given the authority and the credit. The usurping of leadership roles for midwives was perhaps the most important ramification of the move of midwifery toward rationalized school training at the beginning of the twentieth century. This process is illustrated by the example of two schools of midwifery in Milwaukee.

By 1890, the informality of apprentice training had begun to give way to a more structured learning environment. Organized by physicians together with some local midwives, the Milwaukee School of Midwifery and the Wisconsin College of Midwifery offered residents of Milwaukee and other Wisconsin women a potentially more rationalized course of instruction in the theory and the practice of midwifery than they could get by themselves or in tandem with a solo practitioner. Furthermore, these schools offered training close to home: between 1890 and 1907, over half of the Milwaukee Board of Health registrants reported a local school education.

The evolution of midwifery education from informal to formal training paralleled the developments in other helping occupations in this period, and it offered this traditional women's occupation the potential for professional standing. As historians and sociologists have found, education plays a key role in the institutionalization and legitimation of a profession. Historically, instruction for many occupations has evolved from the relative informality of apprenticeships to formal training based on the standardization and codification of knowledge.[35] This standardization provided by a common basis of training is a key indicator used by scholars to measure an occupation's movement towards professionalization. Once established, this school-based education has then been the main support of a professional subculture.[36] In addition to formal training, professional development has also needed to claim an exclusive body of knowledge. To then achieve a monopoly over practice, the profession needs to control both the "production of knowledge and the production of producers," preferably within one institution.[37] In addition, a profession must be free to resolve what Magali Larson and others refer to as the dialectic of the always high ratio between indetermination and technicality.[38] In summary, the professional practitioner must master a body of knowledge unique to the field within a formal setting, and then have the autonomy to decide when and under what circumstances to apply this knowledge.

Many historians of medicine have documented late nineteenth and early twentieth-century medical leaders' attempts to reform medical education and medical licensing. In a response to long-term developments in science and education, medical leaders recognized the need for a multiyear, graded curriculum that included didactic lectures, laboratory work, and supervised clinical instruction. Many small proprietary schools were forced to merge with stronger schools or go out of business. By the beginning of the twentieth century, graduates of medical schools were required to obtain a state-issued license to begin their practice.[39]

But this concern with standardized education and licensure was neither gender specific nor solely a concern of medicine. Turn of the century nursing leaders also called for more training for their practitioners. Schools for nurses, it was believed, would eliminate the natural or "professed" nurse and replace her with a trained professional.[40] Pioneers such as Lucy Walker, superintendent of the Pennsylvania Hospital School for Nurses, and Isabel Hampton, superintendent of the Johns Hopkins Training School, reformed or instituted new nurses' training programs that attempted to teach theoretical science in addition to the traditional practical bedside nursing.[41] By the early twentieth century a few nursing leaders were moving beyond Walker and Hampton, advocating collegiate training as a means of gaining professional standards by upgrading the knowledge and standards of nursing practitioners.[42]

By the first decades of the twentieth century, therefore, leaders of two branches of the healing arts recognized clearly that better training fulfilled their goal of professional development. They understood that professionalization meant credentials based on education and licensing standards that would enable practitioners to assert the value to human life of their specialized knowledge and their special skills. At the same time, however, medical and nursing leaders recognized that professionalization enhanced their status and consolidated their authority, securing their agenda for improving the status of their practitioners.[43]

How did the midwifery schools organized at the end of the nineteenth century measure up in terms of these professional ideals? Were they offering formal training as a result of a codification of knowledge in midwifery? Did this standardized training become the main support of a professional subculture for midwives? These schools' curricula, personnel, and philosophy demonstrate that regardless of the new skills they offered their students, the schools were not, nor were they intended to be, a step in promoting the professionalization of midwifery.

Milwaukee physicians and midwives were not alone in starting training schools for midwives in the United States in the last part of the nineteenth century. There had been sporadic attempts at setting up midwifery schools in the United States throughout the nineteenth century, and by the end of the century, many American cities boasted midwifery schools that offered courses to young and middle-aged women. While the quality of the education offered by some of these schools was questionable, all attempted to upgrade both the skills and the image of female birth practitioners. Because many of the founders of these schools had trained in Europe, it is useful to examine the curricula and the philosophy behind the European schools.

By the middle of the nineteenth century, many European countries boasted of their high-quality midwifery training schools. These institutions, usually associated with a lying-in hospital and the clinic of a university medical department, offered the latest instruction in medical and obstetrical science. For example, Dr. Joseph Spath, a protégé of the great pathologist Dr. Johann Klein, became director of the Midwife Clinic School at Vienna in 1864. He publicly and exclusively adapted Semmelweiss's theory of the causes of puerperal fever.[44] The German Royal School for Midwives at Munich, admired by both British and American observers, had a rigorous course emphasizing aseptic and antiseptic techniques and a thorough understanding of normal and pathological labor.[45]

Entrance requirements for these schools stipulated moral as well as academic qualifications. Applicants were required to have an elementary school education or to pass an examination covering elementary school subjects. Successful applicants in Germany were expected not only to be educated, but also to be mature women "of good character." Even an applicant's class circumstances played a role. German schools gave precedence to the widows of civil officers "in order that they [might] not become a burden on the government."[46] However, a midwifery student needed some family support to pay for her schooling, and this fact probably excluded the poorest women from obtaining training. Most students in all of the European schools paid tuition, the equivalent of $65 to $150 in Germany and up to $200 in France.[47]

The period of instruction in the continental midwifery schools varied from one to two years. Students learned anatomy, physiology, and elementary pathology as well as practical midwifery, often training alongside medical students.[48] A chief midwife instructor might then offer a separate midwifery theory course. To graduate, a pupil midwife usually took an oral examination in front of her teacher and the members of a government commission.

Passing the final examinations was an important step, for by the end of the nineteenth century, many European governments kept a very close watch on their midwives. Often only graduates of the hospital schools were allowed a license to practice, and in some countries midwives were required to take periodic refresher courses.[49]

European midwives and physicians emigrating to the United States took their ideas about training with them. In Milwaukee, older foreign-trained midwives tended to be graduates of the German schools, while later arrivals were more likely to have received diplomas from one of the Austro-Hungarian schools or even a Polish school.[50] Literate, educated, and proud, they sometimes were quite critical of unlicensed, unskilled American midwives. As Agnes Pradzinska, a Milwaukee midwife, wrote in 1896 to *The American Midwife:*

I wish to express my concern that the so-called butcher-women be prohibited. I have already complained many times to the local health department, but I always receive the same answer: "We will look into the matter." But they are still looking into it. The births should all be registered in the State of Wisconsin; such female bunglers don't do it though; among [the female bunglers] is one, who calls herself a midwife and has hung out a shield with the inscription "Midwife and birth assistant." But she can neither read nor write . . . [She] also knows fortune-telling, because when she performs a delivery, she tells the mother how many more children she will have; even better yet is that she also knows how many boys and girls she will have.[51]

A few American schools offering midwifery instruction attempted to give their students an education equal to the best European institutions. The Bellevue Hospital School for Midwives, perhaps the best known American midwifery school in the early twentieth century, opened in New York City in 1911. Unlike most American schools, but in the tradition of the continental ones, the Bellevue school received government financing from the city of New York. Successful applicants had to be between the ages of twenty-three and thirty-five, "cleanly in their person and homes, and of high moral character."[52] Instruction, board, and lodging were provided at no cost, and students lived at the hospital for the entire seven-month course. The resident obstetrician and the nurse superintendent instructed the pupil midwives, who learned to deliver babies both at the hospital and in the community. Each student witnessed at least one hundred confinements and delivered twenty cases on her own, including a large number of primiparas.[53] Graduation and a diploma followed a successful grade on both a written and an oral examination, administered by the visiting obstetrician.[54]

The quality of most American midwifery schools probably varied tremendously, most falling somewhere between the Bellevue Hospital School and the Chicago school where, it was reported, the physician-instructor, often drunk, gave a few lectures in his back office and charged $100 in tuition.[55] This variability could be directly traced to the entrepreneurial character of medical instruction in general in the late nineteenth century. Like many contemporary medical schools, most American midwifery schools were profit-making ventures not associated with hospitals. Sharing the same problems that often plagued proprietary medical schools, many midwifery colleges suffered from poor facilities, insufficient instructional materials, and course work that was made up solely of didactic lectures.

These schools attracted primarily literate young and middle-aged immigrant women accustomed to the legal necessity of training in order to obtain a license to practice.[56] To cater to these immigrant women, many American schools offered their course in both English and another language, usually German.[57] The Deutiche Hebammen

Schule, established in Chicago in 1889, even offered "a parallel course
... in the Swedish language, the only one in America," in addition to
its German-language course.[58]

American midwifery schools developed from and found their roots
in communities like Milwaukee, which were experiencing an enormous expansion of their immigrant communities. As millions of European immigrants poured into the United States between 1880 and
1910, Milwaukee in particular experienced an explosive growth in its
population: in each five-year interval between 1880 and 1900, the
population increased an average of 29 percent. From 1900 through
1910, the rate slowed to a still high 14.5 percent.[59] Much of this
growth was related to immigration from the Old World: between
1880 and 1910, the city was tied for first place among all American
cities in percentage of foreign stock. By 1910, the total foreign stock—
defined as total foreign-born population plus natives with at least one
foreign-born parent—was 78.6 percent of the total population, more
than half German.[60]

As these communities grew, it was not surprising to find many
practicing midwives and midwifery schools based on the European
model. While many of the women who were part of the resurgence
of midwifery in Milwaukee between 1875 and 1910 had been trained
in Europe, the majority of foreign-born midwives were not educated
there. Only 145 (24.6 percent) of the total number of registrants in
the Milwaukee Health Department file attended European schools,
and they represented only 29.1 percent of the school-trained group.
Though large numbers of midwives registered in the 1880s and 1890s,
the number of foreign-trained women dropped from 56.1 percent in
the period 1877–1881 to as low as 11.4 percent in the period 1897–
1901 (see Table 1.1).

The majority of Milwaukee's new midwives in the late nineteenth
century received their education at one of the two midwifery schools
established there in the late 1870s and the 1880s. Both the Milwaukee
School of Midwifery, founded in 1879 by Wilhelmine Stein, a
German-trained immigrant, and the Wisconsin College of Midwifery,
organized by three physicians in 1885 and later run by Mary Klaes, a
German immigrant but American-trained midwife, produced many
graduate midwives for the approximately two decades each school
was in business. Of the 373 women who registered with the state after

Table 1.1   Midwife registrants, Milwaukee Health Department, 1877–1907

Year(s)	School-trained Europe	School-trained Milwaukee	Total school-trained	Total registered
1877–1881	37 56.1%	20 30.3%	66	87
1882–1886	25 37.9%	37 56.1%	66	80
1887–1891	21 27.3%	59 76.6%	77	93
1892–1896	17 13.8%	103 83.7%	123	132
1897–1901	9 11.4%	65 82.3%	79	86
1902–1906	13 32.5%	23 57.5%	40	47
1907	23 48.9%	23 48.9%	47	63

Source: Physicians' Register (Midwife File), (June 1877–October 1907). City of Milwaukee Public Health Department Archives Section, Milwaukee Public Library, Milwaukee, Wisconsin.

Notes: "Total school-trained" includes schools other than Europe and Milwaukee. Percentages are of total school-trained.

1909, 132 (35.4 percent) had trained at one of these two local schools. These schools had a statewide influence: the Milwaukee Registry showed 84 graduates of these schools who gave addresses outside the city, perhaps implying that some students came to Milwaukee specifically for their education.[61]

The Milwaukee School of Midwifery opened in 1879 with five students at the home of one of the founders, Wilhelmine Stein. Stein, born in Germany in 1839, had trained at the Midwifery School at Anstedt, Germany, before emigrating to the United States in 1870.[62] Two Milwaukee doctors, Alphonse F. Kalckhoff and Charles Betzell, joined Stein in cofounding the school. Betzell, who had arrived in Milwaukee from Germany just the year before the school opened, trained in medicine at the Ludwig-Maximilian University at Munich, graduating in 1834.[63] Kalckhoff was a native of the United States. Born in Milwaukee in 1851, he had precepted with a local Milwaukee physician and worked three years in a hospital before graduating from the Rush Medical College in Chicago in February 1876.[64]

28

Though Dr. Kalckhoff provided a link between the immigrant and the native-born communities, it is clear that this school drew support from and appealed to Milwaukee's sizable German-speaking community. This association is depicted explicitly in several large advertisements that appeared during the 1890s in Milwaukee's city directory. Each advertisement for Mrs. Stein's school showed a picture of a substantial building with a German text that mentioned the "Hebammen Schule," with two terms per year and the "Privat Entbindungs Institut" (Private Lying-In Institute).[65]

Though school instruction is intended to rationalize a course of training, Mrs. Stein's school, at least in the early years, adopted a more idiosyncratic teaching style. As with apprentice-trained midwives, the length of the course depended on the student. For example, Rosalia Noll noted that she had taken a course of four months from September 1884 to January 1885,[66] while Anna Schreiber recalled that she had a six-month course in the same year.[67] Until the mid-1880s, when Mrs. Stein opened a lying-in hospital at the same address as the school, student midwives had no hospital experience, though they may have assisted Stein informally at her home deliveries.

By 1887, the school's curriculum had changed to include attendance at confinements as well as didactic lectures. Caroline Kueny, an 1887 graduate, stated that she took a course "of 6 months . . . went through 16 confinements and [was] examined by 2 doctors."[68] Indeed, in the succeeding years, it seemed that this school's midwifery curriculum had become similar to that of contemporary nursing schools, where practical work replaced lectures.[69] It appears that Mrs. Stein had expanded her clinical facilities, probably taking in unwed mothers who desired a secluded place to deliver their babies. Thus, later graduates reported having had little actual coursework, but a great deal of midwifery and maternity nursing experience. Sophia Kegel reported that her education in 1888 consisted of a six-month course, with "about 6 lectures per month." She "assisted 'Preceptoress' Mrs. Wilhelmina [*sic*] Stein at her hospital as well as [at] private confinement cases." Kegel wrote that she had spent time in Mrs. Stein's hospital "daily during the course of study."[70]

The school's curriculum changed again in the early years of the twentieth century. By 1902, Wilhelmine Stein expanded the course offerings at her school, and in 1904 she lengthened the school term to nine months. Some graduates now attended lectures on the anatomy and physiology of the female pelvis, the practice of midwifery, and the care of the child, together with nine months of hospital work.[71]

Though physicians who had trained midwives as apprentices had helped to found the school, throughout the years the school was in operation, the pupil midwives worked closely with Mrs. Stein. Indeed, some graduates later referred to the school as "Mrs. Stein's Hospital."[72] The doctors' roles, on the other hand, appear to have been removed from the day-to-day teaching. Instead, the physicians offered some clinical instruction for difficult cases, examined the pupils for the final degree (as was common in Europe), and publicly represented the school at graduation.[73]

Though the doctors associated with the school did not have much of a pedagogic role, their support and status were necessary for the school's reputation and legitimacy. Thus, when Dr. Kalckhoff, one of the founders, left his post of medical examiner in 1883, another German-trained Milwaukee doctor, Charles Schenermann, took his place.[74] By 1900, at least six different physicians, mostly trained in Germany, had served as medical examiners for the school. In return for their services, the schools provided these immigrant physicians with a familiar institution in their new neighborhood, one that offered them a small measure of prestige and, most likely, some needed cash.

The story of Milwaukee's second school of midwifery is very similar to the first, and it reinforces the concept of physician control over midwifery education and the reliance of midwifery on physician goodwill for the running of its schools. It also demonstrates the complex relationship between midwifery and Milwaukee's immigrant community. The Wisconsin College of Midwifery opened in 1885, listing three physicians as its directors. Two of these three doctors, like the ones associated with the Milwaukee School of Midwifery, had trained in Europe.[75] Three years later, in 1888, more German émigré physicians replaced several of the original founders of the Wisconsin College of Midwifery. The school's personnel by this date also included a midwife, Mary Klaes, who had been trained by one of the original founders of the school.[76] Like many schools in other immigrant communities, the Wisconsin College of Midwifery advertised that its course was taught in both German and English.[77]

By 1889, the school had undergone a fundamental reorganization. Mrs. Klaes, together with two other midwives and three new physicians, had reorganized it as the "Wisconsin College of Midwifery and Lying-In Hospital."[78] More than the name had changed, however. Unlike the physicians at Mrs. Stein's school, the physicians at the Wisconsin College of Midwifery were not part of the immigrant community. Instead, most of the physicians who acted at one time or another over the next twenty-five years as President of the Wisconsin College of Midwifery were American-educated practitioners. In addition, many of these American doctors were young men only recently out of medical school.[79]

The relative youth of these physicians undoubtedly was one reason for their agreeing to serve as medical examiners. As new practitioners in a city full of physicians, perhaps these doctors felt that they would benefit from the exposure of being a medical examiner at the midwifery school. Furthermore, the advertising of their name was free. While the doctors lent only their prestige, Mrs. Klaes assumed most of the school's pedagogical duties and its financial burden. From 1889 to at least 1913, she reincorporated the school and hospital several times, but the school remained based in her home. The school must have prospered during the 1890s, for by 1900 it had been moved to a larger structure that Klaes owned outright.[80]

But though later graduates would refer to "Mrs. Clay's [*sic*] school,"[81] Mary Klaes publicly assumed a secondary role. As advertisements in the city directories demonstrate, Klaes's central role in the Wisconsin College of Midwifery and Lying-In Hospital was minimized by her need to attract doctors to hold the title of President of her school. Listing the physician's name first and in bold print, the text of several advertisements urged other doctors to bring their cases to the school's hospital, with the promise that "trained nurses" were "always in attendance."[82] By 1901, the hospital referred to itself as "St. Mary's Private Sanitarium," having "the Best Physicians in charge." Though midwives trained at the institution through at least 1913, the city directory made no mention of it.[83]

Offered in German and in English, the school's curriculum in the

1890s included didactic lectures and much practical work. Students recalled having lectures in "anatomy, biology, and physiology," with "daily recitations or lectures of two hours each."[84] In the early years, students gained practical experience by attending "obstetrical clinics" at least twice per week. By the mid-1890s, however, many graduates reported that much of their entire four- to six-month term was spent working at Mrs. Klaes's maternity hospital.[85] By 1912, Klaes had expanded the school's term to eight or even twelve months and students attended at least twenty-five confinements.[86] Shortly after this date, however, the school went out of business.

The problem the Milwaukee schools experienced in holding on to the "best physicians" is indicative of the larger problems these and other midwifery schools faced in attempting to train "professional" midwives. When the young doctors who had served as medical examiners no longer needed the public exposure the post gave them, they left. But midwives needed school training, and as mature, married women with families, they needed training close to home. As Figure 1.2 demonstrates, most practitioners who registered with the

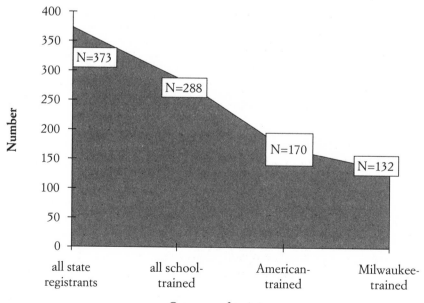

Figure 1.2 Location of midwife training

state had school training. But, as that figure also illustrates, local schools played a crucial role in educating Wisconsin's midwives: Milwaukee-trained midwives constituted almost half of all of the school-trained and as much as 78 percent of the American school-trained practitioners. Clearly, the demise of these schools left women with no place to go to train as midwives.

When the facilities of the Milwaukee School of Midwifery and the Wisconsin College of Midwifery are compared with those of the publicly funded Bellevue Hospital School for Midwives in New York, the Milwaukee schools fall short. But their offerings were at least as good as, if not better than, many other midwifery schools throughout the United States. Indeed, many of Milwaukee's pupil midwives received much more obstetrical training than many American doctors obtained in the medical schools surveyed by J. Whitridge Williams in 1912.[87] Yet no midwifery school helped to promote the professionalization of midwifery.

Midwifery, unlike the other healing arts, claimed neither a distinct body of knowledge nor control over the production of its own practitioners. Many of these problems arose directly from the very schools that might have been expected to build a professional image for their practitioners. Midwifery schools in Europe and in the United States relied heavily on physician cooperation and physician prestige. At the schools in Milwaukee, city physicians gave important lectures and always conducted the final examinations at each school. Thus, even though Mrs. Stein and Mrs. Klaes assumed the financial burdens of their schools and were acknowledged publicly for their leadership roles by their students, they still relied on physicians' decisions as the final authority determining competence. This reliance was typical of midwifery schools throughout the United States. Indeed, an Illinois law went even further in tying midwifery education to the direction of physicians. Passed in 1896, the law required that only "legally qualified" physicians could teach in midwifery schools eligible for state recognition.[88] Furthermore, the prestige of the physician was also critical. Several schools in St. Louis depended upon physician faculty members, and one, the St. Louis School of Midwives, was directed by Dr. George J. Engelmann, who was later to become president of the American Gynecological Society.[89] Both Klaes and Stein recognized doctors' crucial roles in their repeated searches for physicians as presidents of their schools. Indeed, the demise of both schools in the first decades of the twentieth century was undoubtedly linked to their founders' advanced age and their ongoing difficulty at finding cooperative physicians.[90]

In addition to not providing any leadership roles for midwives, midwifery schools reinforced and institutionalized dependence on physicians. Because midwifery could not claim a separate, distinct curriculum apart from obstetrics, student midwives learned that good midwives attended only normal, uncomplicated births. This limitation of the midwife's autonomy was institutionalized in midwifery education in Europe. As an American physician studying midwifery schools in Scandinavia noted approvingly, students "are taught to revere the physician, and they are distinctly shown their limitations."[91] American schools followed this philosophy, as a physician associated with the Bellevue School explained: "Not the least advantage of our primitive attempt to educate the midwife at the Bellevue School is the thorough teaching of each candidate for graduation her limitations . . . one important fact is instilled into the brain of each midwife, and that is the knowledge of her own limitations—the knowledge of what not to do, and when to seek the aid of a practising physician."[92] Although Milwaukee physicians left no written records recording their feelings about the midwifery schools they dealt with, it is reasonable to assume, given their standing in the medical community, that they concurred with the statement issued by a St. Louis school, which insisted, "We shall graduate *Midwives* who are competent to conduct natural labor cases and will not go beyond this . . . We shall *not* graduate female physicians or women who will in any way dabble in medicine."[93]

The lack of leadership roles for midwives in their schools led to further problems for the development of midwifery as a profession. In nursing and in medicine in the early twentieth century, school training led to the development of an elite group who helped to establish sets of credentials for their emerging disciplines. Lacking a nucleus of leaders who could articulate a coherent philosophy of practice, midwifery ceded control to physicians, who then appropriated the responsibility of setting up and administering tests of midwifery competence. Thus, a Wisconsin statute enacted in 1909 was typical of many American and European laws governing midwifery practice.

The statute placed midwifery under the control of the State Board of Medical Examiners with no midwife representation. Even masseurs, placed under the control of the Board in 1916, managed to have their own representatives appointed to serve with the committee overseeing regulation of their craft.[94]

Though some scholars have cited gender as the reason for physicians' contempt for midwives, gender alone does not explain midwives' lack of professional development.[95] Nurses, who faced questions about their own professionalism, also supervised or trained midwives, but they demonstrated little solidarity with these other women. Perhaps as an attempt to bolster their own professional status, nurses, like physicians, berated midwives as dirty and ignorant, and midwifery as an unsafe practice. Paradoxically, though school education was used to professionalize nursing, nurses failed to acknowledge that training could do the same for midwives. Florence Swift Wright, for example, who supervised midwives for the New Jersey State Department of Health reported disdainfully on Mrs. B., an apprentice-trained midwife: "[She] showed a very good knowledge of the duties of a midwife, a love of the work, interest in her poorer neighbors and real *nursing* ability which is often lacking in the sometimes unduly mercenary, trained midwife" (emphasis mine).[96]

This tension between nurses and trained midwives in many cases may have been rooted in the class and ethnic differences between these two women's occupations. Nurses may also have been worried that midwives would compete with them for patients. At least four women who registered for Wisconsin midwife licenses also reported having had nursing training in Europe or the United States. Midwife Ida Hill, for example, reported that she had trained at the Battle Creek Sanitarium for three years, and that her course had included "thorough training . . . [in the] preparations for and process of labor, care of infant, and management of the lying-in."[97] Clara Bogenschild, a Milwaukee midwife, reported that in addition to her midwife training, she had been a nurse in a clinic in Germany for two and a half years.[98] Undoubtedly, some of these midwives eventually abandoned their own craft to do obstetrical nursing.[99]

Midwifery in the United States in the late nineteenth century faced a crisis of professionalism that related directly to the natural evolution of the occupation. As with the other healing arts, formal education displaced apprenticeships, which had, in turn, supplanted the neighbor women's empirical training. Unlike the other branches of medicine, however, each stage of this developmental process for midwives more strictly circumscribed their autonomy to practice. Apprenticed midwives, receiving more systematic training than the casual learning obtained by neighbor women, were most certainly instructed to call physicians for a birth problem, especially if a physician was their mentor. Formal training only reinforced this proscription, leaving graduate midwives mere "birth technicians" who had to rely on real professionals to stay in practice.[100]

In short, school training added problems to midwives' crisis of professionalism. Midwife technicians, always dependent on others to remain in business, now had to rely wholly on professionals in other fields to judge their competence. The professional investigator could then question the fitness of the technician's class, gender, or ethnic background, or even decide that the work itself was inappropriately complex for the technician to handle.

Between 1870 and 1920, the evolution in midwifery training dramatically affected midwives' autonomy to practice. But as the period unfolded, the class, ethnicity, and marital status of midwives posed even more restrictions on the growth of this occupation.

CHAPTER TWO

A Married Woman's Occupation

🦋

When Dora Larson applied for a midwife license with the state of Wisconsin in 1914, she noted that her qualifications for practice included being the mother of eight children and the grandmother of four. Larson also implicitly recorded her ideas about midwifery on her license application, pointing out that she had "lived here in this township 58 years." A Norwegian immigrant who lived on a small farm with her husband in rural southern Wisconsin, Larson wrote that she had attended ninety-five births herself, but that she "never counted where I helped."[1]

Larson's parental and immigrant status was not unusual for midwives. Emilie Roller, to take another example, was a German immigrant midwife who lived in Milwaukee's west side with her artisan husband and her two young children. Despite her family responsibilities, Roller was a very active Milwaukee practitioner, sometimes attending up to twenty-one births a month.[2]

Larson's and Roller's childbearing experiences were typical of Wisconsin's midwives. Almost every midwife practicing in the state also had children, making motherhood seem almost a requirement for the job. Furthermore, Larson and Roller, in addition to their family status, shared two other distinctive characteristics with most Wisconsin midwives: almost all had been born in Europe or had parents who were immigrants, and the overwhelming majority were members of working-class families.

Midwifery was women's work, and regardless of how a midwife was educated, she practiced within a context circumscribed by gender, class, and culture. Thus, the practice of midwifery in the late nineteenth and early twentieth centuries cannot be explained in purely economic terms. Instead, midwives' ethnic status and the gendered expectations of immigrant women about childbirth help to explain which women were called to deliver babies and explain in large part why midwifery remained a traditional occupation of married women. Immigrant, working-class midwives, taking cases based on the needs of their own families, practiced midwifery in a much different way from physicians who attended childbirth. Even trained midwives delivered babies within the traditional confines of their families and their communities rather than adopting the more modern, professional model of the twentieth-century physician. Thus, the relationship between immigrant communities and the practice of midwifery is the key to understanding why midwifery never attained, or was intended to attain, professional status in the health-care hierarchy of the United States.[3]

Midwives and Other Female Healers

At the end of the nineteenth century, women could be found practicing medicine, nursing, and midwifery. But midwives' family ties, class, and ethnicity distinguished them from other female health-care practitioners. These social and cultural differences ultimately set midwifery apart from the professional aspirations of medicine and nursing.

Female physicians came predominantly from middle-class, native-born families. In the years before 1880, most came from the northeast, many from reform-minded Quaker families. By 1900, more women doctors came from the midwest and west as schools in these areas began to create places for female students. Some women doctors were the daughters of physicians, and by the late nineteenth century a few women were even the second generation of female physicians in their families.[4] While a family background in medicine was not essential to success, young women did rely on the financial and emotional support of their families in order to attend school and then to set up a practice.

The costs of medical training required at least a middle-class financial backing. Estimates of the cost of medical school in the nineteenth century ranged from $600 to $2,000, and some students received scholarships to support themselves. Though a few prominent immigrant women found patrons willing to help pay their medical school tuition, most female medical students came from families affluent enough to afford the costs of schooling. Indeed, Dr. Ann Preston, the president of the Pennsylvania Female Medical College in the 1860s, believed that the combination of time and money discouraged the majority of interested young women from pursuing a career in medicine.[5]

Female doctors paid another price in addition to tuition. Many women doctors found that the exigencies of practice seemed to preclude marriage and children. An 1881 survey of women medical school graduates, for example, found that only 15 percent of them had married. Though the numbers of married women doctors did start to rise by the end of the nineteenth century, estimates are that by 1900 only about one-third of female doctors in practice had wed.[6] Professional identity seemed incompatible with the expectations of women as wives and mothers.

Nursing, in some instances, may have represented an alternative to medical school. Young nursing students in America shared many characteristics of women physicians. They too were predominantly white, native-born and the daughters of middle-class families from small towns or rural areas. For example, a study of students at the elite Pennsylvania Hospital School of Nursing revealed that most of its nursing students were young women from small towns who had at least attended high school; many had even more education.[7] Like women physicians, the vast majority of nurses were white. Even as late as 1920, only 3 percent of trained nurses were black, though black women made up 24 percent of the female working population that year.

For many women, however, nursing education may have provided a means for upward mobility. Nurses who attended the more typical schools did not share the genteel social background of women in medicine or law, but they did "represent an elite among working women."[8] For example, most of the women who attended small, non-elite nursing schools in Boston had earned wages at working-class occupations prior to nursing school.[9] Yet, though these women understood that attendance at these more humble schools would keep them from the prestigious assignments after graduation, they still saw nursing as a boost into the middle class.[10]

Whatever the initial class origins of nursing students, the ideology of nursing remained rooted in the middle-class ideal of female service. Students learned this important value as they trained. Throughout the late nineteenth and early twentieth centuries, nursing schools focused on molding their young charges into respectable, middle-class ladies suitable for employment as private duty nurses in the homes of the middle and upper classes.[11] The best nurses were considered to be those who were attractive young women in their twenties and, at least before 1920, most white nurses left the field when they married.[12]

Though by the early twentieth century midwifery, like nursing, increasingly emphasized school training, even graduate midwives shared few demographic or social characteristics with nurses or female physicians. Midwives' age, birthplace, class, and marital status differentiated them from other female health-care practitioners. These demographic characteristics undoubtedly were connected to the way midwifery was practiced and the traditional position it held within the women's community. When a midwife was called to deliver a baby, she would go for a day or an evening. As the director of a group of the parturient woman's neighbors and women family members, the midwife stayed until the baby was delivered and the mother was resting comfortably.[13] A nurse on a case, however, stayed away from home longer, working alone in a patient's house for many weeks at a time. Physicians, male and female, found that the practice of medicine was constant and mostly full time. Given the resulting conflicts between family and occupation, almost all nurses practiced only while they were single, and many women physicians found that they could or would not combine commitments to family and career.[14] Midwifery, on the other hand, allowed a place for married women with families to practice their skills and to earn some money.[15]

Midwives and Their Families

My analysis of 893 Wisconsin midwives found that midwifery students and practitioners were usually immigrant, working-class, middle-aged, married women. A linkage of 398 of these women and their families to their appearance in one of the federal or Wisconsin state manuscript censuses permitted an in-depth analysis of the details of midwife family life.

Each midwife was linked to the first census where she could be found. The data included each midwife's age, her county and city of residence, her birthplace, her marital status, her literacy, the number and ages of her children present in the household, the structure of her household (i.e., whether relatives or boarders lived with her nuclear family), her home ownership status, and the occupation of the head of the household (usually her husband). Table 2.1 gives the breakdown by census year and by county.[16]

With the high rates of immigration to Milwaukee and the rest of Wisconsin in the late nineteenth and early twentieth centuries, it is not surprising to find a strong correlation between a European place of birth and the practice of midwifery. Indeed, the number of midwives practicing in Milwaukee began to rise at the end of the nineteenth century as the number of European immigrants swelled the city. This point did not go unnoticed, as a *Milwaukee Sentinel* article noted in 1889: "No city in the country has as many practicing midwives as Milwaukee, it is said, at least in proportion to population. There are only a comparatively few more physicians than midwives, there being 171 of the former and 115 of the latter."[17]

Figure 2.1, which depicts both the total number of midwives who advertised in the Milwaukee city directory as well as the number of new midwives for each year, shows that the *Sentinel's* observations were not unfounded. In 1870, only fourteen midwives listed themselves in the city directory; by 1900, there were 171. Furthermore, the market was quite fluid. Until 1905, many new practitioners entered

Table 2.1 Midwives by census year and by county

Census year	Number	County	Number
1870	6	Milwaukee	301
1880	77	Dane	33
1900	191	Trempealeau	26
(1905)	38	Price	38
1910	86		
Total	398		398

Sources: 1870, 1880, 1900, 1910 United States and 1905 State of Wisconsin Manuscript Census Schedules for Milwaukee, Dane, Trempealeau, and Price counties.

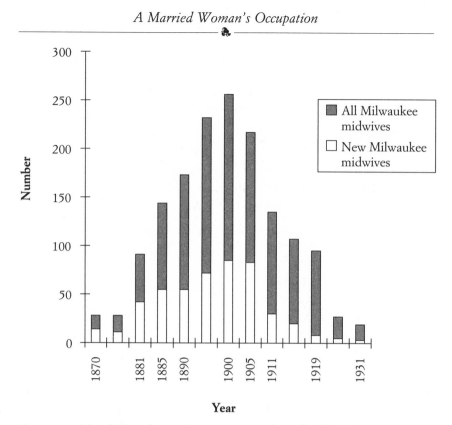

Figure 2.1 New Milwaukee midwives compared to all Milwaukee midwives, 1870–1931

the market even as many others left. In fact, between fifty-five and eighty-five new midwives began their practice within each five-year period between 1885 and 1905.[18]

Given the high numbers of midwives arriving in Milwaukee during the peak years of immigration to the city, it should not be surprising to find that the overwhelming majority of midwives traced in the census were immigrants. Most of the midwives in the Wisconsin census sample were first-generation immigrants, and all but ten had parents born in Europe (see Figure 2.2). With the high percentage of German immigrants in Wisconsin, the majority of these women, not surprisingly, came from Germany (53 percent). Indeed, the German-speaking midwives, including those born in Germany, Austria-Hungary and Switzerland, constituted over 60 percent of all of the foreign-born women in the sample. The next largest groups of

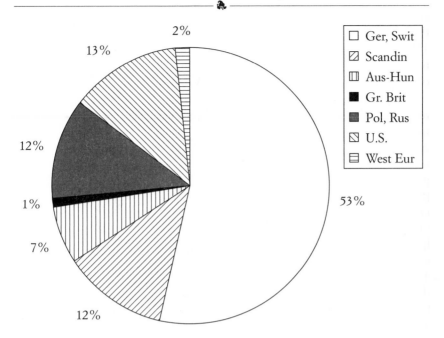

Figure 2.2 Birthplace of Wisconsin midwives located in census (1870, 1880, 1900, 1905, 1910) (*n* = 398)

foreign-born attendants were Polish and Russian, and Scandinavian, each at around 12 percent.

Wisconsin's high percentage of immigrant midwives was not unusual. Historians of midwifery in the United States have long noted the high percentage of midwives who were immigrant women,[19] and many contemporary studies linked these birth attendants to ethnic communities. As Michael Davis noted in his 1921 study of immigrant health, "The immigrant mother has rarely been accustomed to a man doctor at the time of confinement. She and her friends have used the midwife, who, in most European countries, is a woman of some standing, trained, and in many countries carefully supervised. The midwife is the most important single element in the general question of the care of immigrant mothers."[20] Florence S. Wright, a public health nurse supervising New Jersey midwives, even saw a role for midwives in helping to "Americanize" their neighbors.[21]

Contemporary critics of midwives, usually physicians, also commented often on these women's immigrant status. For example, Joseph B. DeLee, a vocal and often vitriolic opponent of midwives, noted approvingly in 1915 that midwives seemed to be relegated to "crowded communities of foreigners."[22] James Lincoln Huntington's survey of midwives in Massachusetts found at least 150 midwives in the state, primarily based "in the manufacturing cities of about 100,000 population, largely composed of immigrants." In Boston, he found that many of the midwives were Italian women, "in the prime of life," who lived in "fairly good homes."[23]

Despite Huntington and DeLee's conclusions, "communities of foreigners" were not restricted only to crowded urban areas. Indeed, immigrant midwives could be found in rural as well as urban areas. A 1924 study of Minnesota midwives found that over half of the state's midwives practiced in rural areas, and most of these practitioners lived in counties with large foreign-born populations. Only 13.7 percent of the midwives in this survey were born in America, while 86.3 percent (101 of 117 midwives) were foreign-born.[24] A Children's Bureau study of maternity conditions in a northern rural Wisconsin county published in 1919 found that the large number of German and Polish settlers clung to "their foreign customs and habits of thought and to a certain extent to their languages, making the district as a whole distinctly foreign in its atmosphere."[25] Midwife attendance at childbirth was one of the "foreign customs" these women "clung to." Twenty-four midwives, all members of the German or Polish communities, practiced in the county, though only a few were reported to be earning their living as midwives. Most of these female attendants were neighbor-women midwives—they "went out" as an accommodation to their neighbors. Of all of the midwives in the region, only six practitioners delivered more than ten babies per year, and only two oversaw more than thirty.[26]

As this Children's Bureau study suggests, Wisconsin midwives practiced not only in cities but also in rural areas where there were significant communities of immigrants. In fact, I found that in Wisconsin, American-born midwives were a distinct minority. While Milwaukee had fewer American-born midwives than expected (the expected number was 39.3; the actual was only 30), the number of American-born midwives in the other three counties in my study were so small that statistical analysis was not feasible.[27] Tests of significance showed distinct ethnic groupings in each county, with Scandinavians predominantly in the three rural areas and Polish and Russian mid-wives exclusively in Milwaukee.

In Milwaukee county, only 7.6 percent of 301 birth attendants were born in America. The overwhelming majority, 185 (61.5 percent), had come from Germany. The three other, predominantly rural, counties showed a similar pattern, though the dominant ethnic group was not always German. In Dane county, only 6 of 33 midwives were native-born. As in Milwaukee, Dane County had a large number of German-born midwives (15, or 45.5 percent), but Scandinavian attendants were almost as numerous (10, or 30.3 percent). In Price and Trempealeau counties, about one-fifth of the practicing midwives were born in the United States. In these two very rural counties, Scandinavian women were the dominant ethnic group. Over 65 percent (n = 17) of the female birth attendants in Trempealeau County were from Scandinavia, and in Price County, 13 women (34.2 percent) were born in Norway, Sweden, or Denmark. In addition, 5 midwives in Price County were natives of Finland.

Besides their immigrant status, other factors delineated the unique characteristics of female birth attendants such as Dora Larson and Emilie Roller. As working, married women, both they and other Wisconsin midwives were part of the small minority of wage-earning housewives at the turn of the twentieth century. Yet, as trained midwives, their credentials for their job set them apart from most other working mothers even as their family situations differentiated them from other health-care workers. Midwives, were, after all, working mothers in an era when most married women did not work outside the home for cash wages. The social and economic dimensions of midwife family life provides a context for explaining both how and why midwives practiced their craft, and they suggest that midwives were motivated to practice by a complex intersection of gender and culture.

Midwives were, above all, married women, and the information on marital status from the census underscored this traditional relationship. Of the 394 women whose marital status could be determined, 316 (80.2 percent) were married women living with their husbands. Another 59 women (15 percent) were widowed, and 11 midwives were divorcées. Only 8 midwives (2.0 percent) were women who had never married. For midwives in Wisconsin, as elsewhere, matrimony remained an unwritten, but almost required, prerequisite for the job.

Determining the actual age of practicing midwives is crucial in understanding both how midwifery was practiced and why it did not last in the United States. Both historians and early twentieth-century observers have claimed that midwives were women of advanced years and that "advanced age" played a role in the demise of midwifery.[28] This assessment, however, overlooks one key point about midwifery—that is, that midwifery has always been an occupation for mature, married women. Since many midwives traditionally learned their craft from observing other midwives and from their own births, it is logical to assume that many people equated expertise with experience and age. Furthermore, since childbirth was the outcome of a sexual encounter, usually only mature women were welcome in the birth chamber. In fact, young single women often were not allowed to become midwives. The career of Dr. Marie Zakrzewska, the director of the New England Hospital for Women, illustrates this stricture. As a young woman, prior to her arrival in America, she had trained to be a midwife in one of the most prestigious schools in Berlin. Her acceptance to the German school was not easy, however. Even with influential support, her first application for admission was refused specifically because she was not married and because at age eighteen she was considered too young to be a midwife.[29]

Midwives needed to be mature women, but they were not superannuated. Most Wisconsin midwives were women in their forties. Among the 373 women who registered after 1909 for a state midwife license, the mean age was about 48 years. Many women from this group were even younger—the school-educated practitioners were significantly younger.[30] Because my census study traced midwives to the first census where they could be found, it identified practitioners earlier in their careers than did the midwife licenses. Thus, the mean age of the 398 midwives found through the census was 43.9, a mean that did not change significantly between 1870 and 1910.[31] Less than 10 percent of midwives in the census study were over the age of sixty (see Figure 2.3).

As might be expected, age did vary by marital status. The census sample was heavily weighted towards married women living with their husbands, and the mean age of these women was 42.66. The 59 wid-

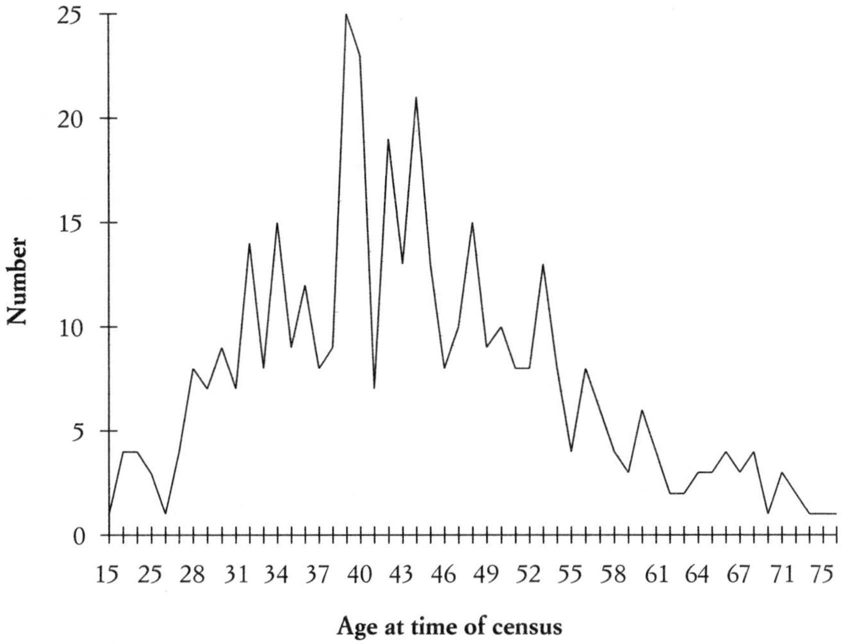

Figure 2.3   Age distribution of midwives from census (1870, 1880, 1900, 1905, 1910) (*n* = 398)

owed practitioners were significantly older than the married or divorced, with a mean age of 51.83. The few single women were significantly younger than either the married or the widowed midwives. Their mean age was 31.25 with a large standard deviation of 9.19.[32]

Like many other working women in their community, midwives left their homes in order to earn money to help support their families. As married women, however, their work-force participation placed them in a unique category of working women. Historians have found that few married women, even immigrant women, ever left home to participate in the wage labor force. In Europe, as industrialization advanced, fewer married women worked outside the home for cash wages.[33] In the United States, as late as 1930, a married woman who had children and who worked outside of the home was a signal that the family was in dire economic straits.[34]

Midwifery, therefore, should be regarded within this domestic context. Indeed, the census data suggest that although the educational process for training midwives had moved outside of the home and family to a formalized setting, the constituency from which midwifery drew its practitioners did not change. An analysis of husbands' occupations, the ages of children, and midwives' own ages reveals that even as midwives had little in common with other female healers, they also did not share common characteristics with women who left the home to perform wage work. Thus, though midwives undoubtedly valued the monetary return from their practice, the particular demographic characteristics of midwives suggest that these women "caught babies" for reasons beyond the sheer need to make money. As in eighteenth-century America or Europe, midwifery remained a particular kind of "women's work."[35]

In the industrializing economies of the late nineteenth century, only married women whose husbands were employed in very low status jobs left the home to perform wage labor. The husbands of Wisconsin's midwives, however, were not predominantly at the bottom of the occupational ladder. Instead, of the 314 husbands whose occupation could be traced, most were skilled artisans (42 percent or 131). The next largest occupational groups were much smaller: 17.2 percent (54) of midwife spouses worked on farms or in the lumber or fishing trade, and 16.9 percent (53) worked as laborers. (See Figure 2.4 for the complete distribution.)[36]

These ratios varied somewhat by ethnic group. An analysis of midwives' birthplace by husbands' occupations shows more skilled artisans among German midwife families than would be expected (100 actual families, while only 76 would be expected). On the other hand, slightly more Polish midwife families were headed by unskilled laborers than would be expected (19 actual versus 15 expected). Not surprisingly, given their almost exclusively rural residence, most of the husbands of Scandinavian midwives were farmers.[37]

Though they eschewed wage work outside the home, working-class married women in western Europe and the United States in the nineteenth and early twentieth centuries did not assume the idealized Victorian role of complete economic dependence and idealized femininity. Indeed, peasant and laboring families in Europe expected all family members to contribute to the survival of the family unit. In the United States, many married women contributed to their family's economy through work that could be performed within the home.

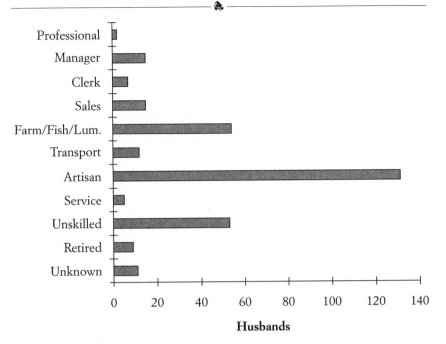

Figure 2.4 Midwives' husbands' occupations from census (1870, 1880, 1900, 1905, 1910) ($n = 314$)

Keeping boarders and lodgers, doing piecework or laundry, and performing other work at home enabled married women to contribute to the family economy and still take care of the family's and the household's needs. Like midwifery, these tasks represented the commercialization of women's traditional domestic skills.[38]

Keeping boarders was perhaps the most popular way for married women to supplement the family income at the turn of the century. In Chicago in 1920, for example, nearly half of those classified in the census as working married women earned their money by keeping lodgers.[39] Families took in boarders in part because it provided a flexible schedule and income for work performed by the wife within the home.[40] Furthermore, keeping boarders fit within the cultural expectations of many ethnic groups about the proper place for married women. In Italian communities, for example, married women rarely held paid employment, but they frequently housed lodgers.[41]

Midwifery, like keeping boarders and lodgers, was in many ways an ideal occupation for mature married women. Though midwives worked outside their own home, they delivered babies in other women's homes, thus remaining protected from the popularly accepted ill effects of the shop floor. Furthermore, just as women who kept boarders could adjust their job schedule to meet the needs of their families, midwives could take fewer cases if they needed time at home or more cases if they needed extra money. Indeed, when viewed in the context of home-based wage earning, midwifery may have replaced keeping boarders. Only 31 midwife families in the census study (7.8 percent) also had boarders present. Instead, most midwife families were nuclear: 287 midwives (72.1 percent) lived with only their husband and children. These numbers did not vary by the midwife's own birthplace or by her social class.[42]

The percentage of families with boarders is significantly low when midwife families are compared to families sharing similar ethnic and class backgrounds and age distributions. John Modell and Tamara Hareven's study of New England families, for example, found percentages of boarders as high as 60 percent in immigrant, working-class families where the head of the household and his wife were in their forties.[43] However, when comparing midwifery and taking in boarders, it must be remembered that keeping lodgers in one's home did not require special training or licenses from the health authorities.

The care of children historically (and even now) has often limited married women's potential for work outside the home, and many Wisconsin midwives were responsible for their own minor children even as they were on call to deliver other women's babies. In the census study, 323 midwives had at least one child living at home with them (83.5 percent). Many women had more: the mean number was about three. The range was quite narrow, however, as most practitioners (77 percent) had four or fewer children at home.[44] Married, divorced, or widowed women did not have significantly different numbers of children.[45]

The mean age of midwives' children also differentiated midwives from those mothers who typically were forced to perform wage work. In most cases, if a mother was compelled to find employment outside of the home, she worked only when her children were very young, and she stopped working when they reached the age of nine or ten, an age when their wages could replace hers.[46] The mean age of midwives' oldest children, 16.0, and the mean age of the youngest, 8.1, deviated considerably from this pattern.[47]

While industrial work for mothers was linked to the number and ages of children, and thus to these children's wage-earning potential, midwifery practice was independent of both these factors. Indeed, a multivariate analysis of effect of the number of children and their ages on midwife practice provided more evidence for looking beyond the economic considerations of midwifery practice. In a multiple regression analysis of 274 midwives found in both the census study and in the birth records, no relationship was found between the number of babies a midwife delivered and the number of her own children, the age of her oldest, or the age of her youngest child. A very weak relationship did exist between the size of a midwife's practice and her age.[48] These findings, together with the mean age of midwives themselves, indicate that midwives began their practice when their children reached school age, and it implies that midwives were not forced by monetary considerations alone to take up their craft.

Even the figures on home ownership among midwife families did not provide convincing evidence of midwifery's particular economic incentive. In the nineteenth century, home ownership was a very slow and expensive process. Amortizing mortgages, common to today's home buyers, were rare. Working-class families were required, therefore, to save a large sum of money to pay off the principal at the end of the loan period, even as they paid the interest in semiannual payments.[49] Of the 320 midwife families whose housing status could be verified, 47 percent rented their homes (151 families), 29 percent held mortgages (92), and 24.1 percent (77) owned their homes outright. Thus, over half of midwives' families were involved in home ownership, a figure consistent with Thernstrom's findings for working-class families in Newburyport, Massachusetts.[50] Furthermore, an analysis of the size of a midwife's practice showed no statistical connection with the status of her family's house. Midwives with mortgages, therefore, did not work more than midwives who rented or owned their homes outright.[51]

While the desire to buy a home undoubtedly provided some economic incentive for midwives, the other demographic characteristics of Wisconsin's midwives did not fit the model of working mothers in the nineteenth century. Furthermore, as the analysis of midwife practice in Chapters 3 and 4 demonstrates, there was no clear-cut relationship between family status and the size of a midwife's practice. Tests of significance showed no connection for urban midwives between the total number of babies a midwife attended and her husband's occupation. Poorer practitioners were not more active than those who might be better off. Midwives married to day laborers were not significantly more active practitioners than midwives married to men who had higher-status occupations such as carpentry or clerking. As would be expected, however, place of practice did make a significant difference. Rural midwives, married mostly to farmers, delivered significantly fewer babies than did urban midwives.[52]

The Wisconsin data are also consistent with some early twentieth century studies of immigrant midwives. These studies, while sometimes decrying the mercenary aspects of midwifery practice, acknowledged that most immigrant midwives were not dependent for their livelihood on their midwifery practice. A study of Chicago's midwives, for example, inveighed against Italian midwives, who seemed to be profiting from fee splitting with the Italian physicians who supervised them. Yet the authors also noted that "the majority of midwives visited were not dependent on their practice for a livelihood, the husband or grown children contributing largely to the support of the family."[53] James Lincoln Huntington's survey of midwives in Massachusetts also found that most midwives in the state worked only part time. Most midwives in Boston, for example, were "not professional midwives, many of them working without pay for their friends and neighbors. Only six of the seventeen [Boston midwives] cared for more than 20 women a year and not one of them for more than 60 cases."[54]

While much of the evidence about Wisconsin's midwives shows that the demographic profile of midwives did not resemble that of industrial workers, it would be misleading to deny the economic benefits of midwifery practice. But, of course, economic incentive varied by the number of patients a midwife was willing to wait on. As the next chapter details, relatively few of the midwives in the Wisconsin sample had sizable practices. Indeed, a large number of these women delivered only one or two babies. For these midwives, it would be difficult to discern any obvious economic rationale. Some money could be made, however, by those midwives who went beyond the role of helpful neighbor woman. In this case, the economic rationale for midwifery needs to be understood within the context of European immigrants' traditional culture, ideas about gender, and developing American ideas about professionals.

CHAPTER THREE

Neighbor Women in the Country

❦

"The employment of midwives," noted Florence Brown Sherbon and Elizabeth Moore in their 1916 survey of childbearing conditions in rural Marathon County, Wisconsin, "appears to be both a result of isolation in the Wisconsin forests and a survival of European custom." The authors, who were conducting the survey for the Children's Bureau, went on to offer some reasons. "Many foreign women prefer a woman rather than a man to help at childbirth; [and] . . . the neighborhood midwife is easier to secure than the doctor and more likely to be on time for the delivery."[1]

Though many women in this rural county relied on midwives, Sherbon and Moore did not find professional midwives in Marathon County. Only a few made a living from their craft. As in many rural areas, most Marathon County midwives " 'went out' mainly as an accommodation to their neighbors." Indeed, Sherbon and Moore noted, "it frequently happens that one of the neighbor women who are called upon to help in emergencies develops special skill in such work and soon finds herself more and more drafted into service."[2]

Throughout the late nineteenth and early twentieth centuries, midwives in many parts of rural America had much in common with the female birth attendants studied by Sherbon and Moore. Anna Folkedahl and Minnie Schiedt were typical. A Norwegian immigrant, Mrs. Folkedahl had graduated in 1871 from the Fraduate Midwifery School in Bergen before coming to the United States in 1887. By 1900, she was forty-seven years old, living in Trempealeau County in a mortgaged house with her husband, probably a farm laborer, and their six children, who ranged in age from fifteen to twenty-seven years. Her midwifery practice averaged about one birth per month, and by 1917, she reported having delivered over five hundred fifty babies during the course of her forty-six-year practice.[3] Minnie Schiedt was a thirty-four-year-old German immigrant housewife living in Blooming Grove in Dane County. Acting at least once as a midwife, she delivered an in-law's eighth child on May 5, 1900.[4] She never applied for a midwife license, and thus there is no information on her training. Indeed, since Schiedt is not recorded as having attended another birth, it is likely that she did not regard herself in a formal sense as a practicing midwife.

Anna Folkedahl and Minnie Schiedt represented each end of the educational spectrum for midwives. At one end was Anna Folkedahl, a school-trained midwife, who was presumably called out for her knowledge. At the other was Minnie Schiedt, who acted as a midwife only within the confines of her family. Yet in Wisconsin, at least, midwifery education alone did not separate the professional from the occasional practitioner. As Table 3.1 shows, location of practice, whether rural or urban, had a dramatic impact on how often a midwife attended a delivery. Table 3.1 demonstrates the differences between the midwife practice of urban and rural midwives identified from the birth certificates in the four counties of this study. Almost 71 percent of rural midwives delivered an average of fewer than six babies per year, while almost half (47.5 percent) of Milwaukee midwives attended twenty-four or more deliveries a year.[5] Part of the explanation for this dissimilarity lies with the obvious differences be-

Table 3.1 Average annual midwife practice by urban and rural counties

Average deliveries per year (*n*)	Rural (percent)	Urban (percent)
1–6	70.8	17.5
6–12	24.5	14.6
12–24	4.7	20.4
24–48	0.0	28.3
48–125	0.0	19.2

Sources: Sampled birth records, 1870–1920: Birth Records, Milwaukee, Trempealeau, Price Counties, Wisconsin Vital Records Office, Wisconsin Department of Health and Human Services, Madison, Wisconsin (WDHHS); also Birth Records, Dane County, Dane County Vital Records Office (DCVRO).

tween the number of potential patients in urban versus rural Wisconsin. However, population statistics do not provide a full explanation. As Sherbon and Moore found in their study, many midwives were employed in Marathon County, while few female birth attendants practiced in the equally rural areas of Wisconsin's Iowa County. Furthermore, in one village in Marathon County where a doctor practiced, a midwife delivered over one-third of the village babies.[6] Thus, the practice of midwifery has to be considered within its larger social and cultural context. At its core, midwifery was an extension of women's domestic duties, and in the traditional rhythms of rural life, it retained this domestic paradigm.

Even by the late nineteenth century, the life and the work of most people in Trempealeau, Price, and rural Dane County, Wisconsin, remained tied to the seasonal work of agriculture. Rural life was isolated, and though there were a few small villages in these three counties, logging and dairy or grain farming employed most families. Economic rewards were hard won; but, as in most of the midwest, the majority of farmers managed to own their own land.[7] For the vast majority of rural women in Wisconsin, as elsewhere, marriage and children remained at the center of adult life.[8]

Just as they shared demographic characteristics, midwives in these three rural counties undoubtedly also shared their neighbors' social values. Many of these values centered around the nature of men's and women's work. Rural Wisconsin, like many farming areas at the end of the nineteenth century, underwent profound economic change, from subsistence to commodity-based agriculture. Trempealeau County led the state in wheat production, though farming in this area, like others in the state, was in the midst of a change to dairying. Price County first developed as a prime logging area as the railroads moved north, but after 1900, agriculture replaced logging, and the number of farms increased dramatically.[9] For the male members of communities in all these counties, agricultural work was becoming more enmeshed in the wider commercial markets that were expanding nationally and even internationally. Women, however, continued to engage in subsistence work, selling small amounts of butter, eggs, poultry, and goods that might yield petty cash for the household, while their husbands' earnings went to pay for the farm mortgage and other expenses.[10]

Patterns of midwifery practice in sampled rural areas of Wisconsin show that midwifery should be considered within this context of subsistence production. The analysis shows that whatever her educational or even ethnic background, no rural midwife took on large numbers of cases, and most midwives attended women who were confined only in their neighborhood. Midwifery remained part of the gender-specific mutual aid that farm women had provided for one another before the advent of commercial markets.[11]

As Chapter 1 demonstrated, levels of midwife education differed most significantly among Wisconsin's rural midwives. Though some school-educated and apprentice-trained midwives practiced in rural Wisconsin, 34 of the 39 neighbor women who applied for midwife licenses after 1909 lived in rural areas of the state. But the identification of midwives from the birth certificates shows that in the rural and frontier areas of Wisconsin, more unregistered women acted as neighbor-woman midwives, attending a few deliveries in the course of their careers. These women made up a significant proportion of practicing midwives: for over half of the midwives in all three rural counties, no information about them could be found other than their name on one baby's birth certificate.[12] Helping out a neighbor or family member, these untrained, occasional practitioners exemplified midwifery's most traditional, domestic roots.

Mrs. R., a neighborhood midwife in Marathon County who was interviewed for the Children's Bureau study, epitomized the rural neighbor-woman midwife. Born in Germany, Mrs. R. bore three children of her own under the care of a midwife before coming to Wisconsin about 1876. She went on to have eight more children on the farm she and her husband and family claimed through homesteading. Mrs. R. became a neighborhood midwife through her own childbearing experience and by reading a textbook on midwifery that she brought with her from Germany. The interviewers found that she had attended about sixteen births in two years, but that five of these were the births of her own grandchildren. Other neighbors also called upon her, but she appears not to have charged a regular fee for her services.[13]

The concept of neighbor-woman midwife denoted both a lack of education and a very localized practice. Mrs. J. Renz, who lived in rural Dane County, was typical. She assisted her neighbor, Mrs.

Sandven, who lived on the next farm down the road, in December of 1910. Like many neighbor women, she never registered as a midwife, and there are no records of her attending other births.[14] Midwives like Mrs. Renz and Mrs. R. stepped in to help out a relative or a friend when some kind of rudimentary experience was needed and no one else was available.[15] Indeed, of the seventy-two neighbor-woman midwives in the three rural counties, only five were not from the same town as the mothers they delivered.[16]

In some rural areas of the United States, neighbor-woman midwives were the only ones available. Even in the late nineteenth century in the Nanticoke Valley of upstate New York, for example, there were no women who identified themselves as midwives. Instead, older women were called upon to help their younger relatives.[17] In a mountainous county of north Georgia in the 1920s, only one of forty-three midwives interviewed by the Children's Bureau had any formal training. As the author of the Georgia study noted, most of the midwives were "granny women," usually "older women in the various communities who had brought up large families themselves and who had a considerable practice, even if limited to attendance at the births of their grandchildren and great-grandchildren."[18] In rural Montana as well, there were no licensed midwives. In a Children's Bureau study of an unnamed large homesteading county, the researchers found that 122 neighbor women attended 181 confinements. As one mother told the Children's Bureau, "One neighbor does it for another out here."[19]

Though neighbor-woman midwives were in the majority in rural Wisconsin, some trained midwives practiced in Trempealeau, Price, and rural Dane and Milwaukee Counties.[20] Attending midwifery school was obviously one way to differentiate oneself from the casual neighbor woman. Anna Folkedahl, living in Trempealeau County, Amy Semerau, of Price County, and Ottile Lange, of Wauwatosa (a suburb of Milwaukee) trained for a year at schools in Europe. Four other women from Trempealeau and Price Counties who registered for state licenses reported training by apprenticeships to other midwives or to physicians.[21]

Training and registration did not predict active, long-term, practices for rural midwives, however. Mrs. Charles Hjort, of Prentice in Price County, attended twenty-four births in the sampled years between 1888 and 1915. Though she thought of herself as a midwife (she registered with the State Medical Practice Board as a midwife in 1909), Mrs. Hjort's practice was sporadic. She averaged only one or two deliveries a year except for 1895, when she oversaw sixteen births.[22]

Mrs. Hjort's sporadic practice was fairly typical for rural midwives who were not neighbor women. With "active midwives" defined as those who attended more than five sampled births, Figure 3.1 charts the yearly average number of active midwives per county with the mean number of births each active midwife delivered. As Figure 3.1 demonstrates, even so-called active rural midwives did not have especially busy practices. Throughout the period of the study, active rural midwives attended only about eight births per year, or one birth every month and a half. Furthermore, the details provided by Table 3.2 show that this leisurely pace was not necessarily related to length of practice.

Table 3.2 groups active rural midwives by the year they began their practice, and it shows the average maximum number of deliveries attended by each cohort together with the number of midwives in the

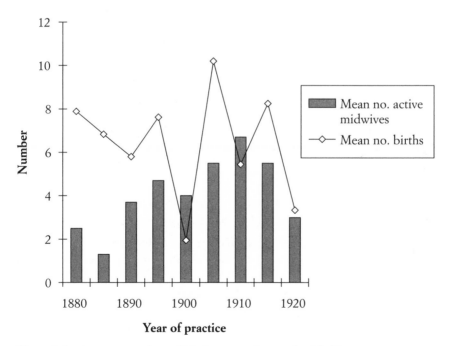

Figure 3.1 Average number of births per active rural midwife

Table 3.2 Active rural midwives in Trempealeau, Price, and rural Dane Counties

Year began practice	No. of midwives	Mean max no. of deliveries	No. of midwives found in successive years
1880	6	7.5	4
1885	1	8.0	0
1890	11	9.0	2
1895	10	7.0	4
1900	9	6.6	8
1905	10	7.5	3
1910	15	5.4	7
1915	4	4.5	2
1920	0	0.0	—

Sources: Sampled birth records, 1880–1920: Birth Records, Milwaukee, Trempealeau, Price Counties, Wisconsin, WDHHS; also Birth Records, Dane County, DCVRO.

cohort who were found practicing in successive years. As the table demonstrates, even at their busiest period, active rural midwives attended fewer than one delivery per month. Furthermore, even this modest activity declined over time. The midwives who began practice in 1910 or 1915 delivered on average fewer than one baby every other month.

Unlike Isabel Larson, who began her practice in Trempealeau County in 1900 and could be found delivering babies as late as 1920, most rural midwives practiced only for a few years.[23] As the figures on the number of midwives found in successive years in Table 3.2 show, many midwives, even active ones, practiced for only a short time. Rachel Berry, for example, who lived in Price County, delivered fifteen babies during 1885 and 1886 and then stopped practicing.[24]

While the concept of the neighbor-woman midwife implies a midwifery practice confined to close relatives or neighbors, female birth attendants who sought training and identification as midwives might have been expected to have attended patients over a wider geographic area. However, whatever their self-identification or training, midwives who practiced in the three rural or frontier counties of this study delivered babies within their own villages or occasionally in a nearby town. One explanation for this limitation might have been the lack of available transportation. As the Children's Bureau study of maternity conditions in northern Wisconsin remarked, "The employment of midwives seems to have been a natural—almost an inevitable—result of the isolation of many of the early settlements and of many neighborhoods at the present day."[25]

Although many rural residents faced formidable problems with transportation, midwifery practice in Wisconsin was not related to the absence of reliable transportation. Though some counties with poor roads and long distances between doctors did have large numbers of midwife-attended births, other counties with similar transportation problems had virtually no midwives practicing in them at all. For example, only two percent of Iowa County's roads were paved, yet almost no births were overseen by midwives. But in similarly rural Marathon County, where five percent of the roads were paved, a midwife attended births in the same village where a doctor also practiced obstetrics.[26]

These patterns of the neighborly location of midwife practice reflected midwifery's ongoing paradigm of domesticity, a paradigm rooted in rural women's traditional perceptions of social obligations and work patterns. The social life of rural farm women, in contrast to men, remained anchored to older forms of kinship and locality. The differences in social life also extended to different perceptions of work among men and women. As historian Nancy Grey Osterud has argued, rural women thought of sharing work in terms of coming to each other's mutual aid, while men increasingly thought of shared work in market terms, even among relatives.[27]

Like rural women's general patterns of sociability and mutual aid, the extent of midwifery practice was delineated by the larger extended family and neighbors regularly visited. Thus, for almost all the rural midwives I studied, the geographic boundaries of their practice corresponded to the political boundaries set by the village and nearby farms. Rather than attending women from all over a county, midwives in rural Wisconsin restricted their practice to the boundaries roughly defined by townships, an area within a county that usually covers about thirty-six square miles.[28]

These geographical limitations on practice held for all the midwives, regardless of their training or their family circumstances. Even Isabel Larson, whose husband was reported as unemployed, confined her midwifery practice within a tight radius of the small farming com-

munity of Whitehall in Trempealeau County. About half of her patients came from her own village, and the rest from nearby farming
communities.[29] Despite Anna Folkedahl's hospital training and the
uncertainty of her husband's farm labor wages, her midwifery practice
was limited almost exclusively to her own village of Ettrick.[30]

Even in sparsely settled areas of Wisconsin, where families lived far
from any other women or medical help, midwives practiced close to
home, regardless of their economic or family circumstances. Mrs.
Charles Hjort was an early resident of Price County, having settled in
this remote logging area after emigrating from Sweden in 1880. With
the influx of young families of childbearing age, demand for maternity
care must have been high, for Mrs. Hjort took up midwifery almost
immediately after an apprenticeship with a local doctor or midwife.
Nonetheless, her midwifery practice remained restricted: of 24 sampled births in 1900, 19 were mothers from her own village.[31] Even
premature widowhood by 1900 did not alter this pattern. Despite the
obvious need for her services in a county with very few physicians,
Mrs. Hjort chose to use her homemaking skills to support herself
and her two small children rather than expanding her midwifery practice. Taking on a boarder, she employed a very traditional strategy of
nineteenth-century female-headed households.

Mrs. Hjort's addition of a boarder to her household may have reflected her inability to support her family on her midwifery earnings.
Just as the sale of butter, eggs, or poultry yielded petty cash, midwives'
fees must have generated only enough money to supplement the family's income. As previously mentioned, neighbor-woman midwives
often received little or no payment for their work. If a delivery was
done for a family member, payment would not be expected.[32] Other
times, these midwives might receive $2 or $3. Though the evidence
is sketchy, it appears that even trained midwives received very little
money for a birth. These midwives did establish regular charges, but
even by 1915, the maximum amount was $5. As an active Polish mid-
wife interviewed in Marathon County explained, "Sometimes [I am
paid] 50 cents, sometimes $2, sometimes $5, sometimes they forget
to pay anything."[33] Another midwife in this county, Mrs. M., ordi-
narily charged $5. Patients' families were expected to provide trans-
portation but, unlike other midwives, Mrs. M. did make twice-daily
visits for nine or ten days after the delivery.[34]

Though women patients in Marathon County reportedly clamored for Mrs. M.'s services, it is doubtful that even she made very much money from her midwifery practice. Based on the evidence from other areas of rural Wisconsin, Mrs. M. probably attended between one and two births per month at the most. If similarly active rural midwives were paid the highest rates for each birth, their total yearly income from midwifery corresponded to the income some farm women reported from their butter and poultry production in the same time periods.[35]

Mary Gerrard's midwifery practice in St. Joseph's Ridge, a farming area outside of LaCrosse, Wisconsin, illustrates this point. She averaged about 28 births per year between 1878 and 1883, and her charges for the years she practiced in this rural area averaged $3 per delivery, for a yearly mean income of $82.50.[36] Her midwifery income was roughly equal to that of farm women who made and sold butter. For example, Guri Olsdatter, a Norwegian farm woman in Minnesota, made an income of $62 from her butter sales during the summer of 1863. This equivalence did not change by the early decades of the twentieth century. Even when rural midwives received $5 per birth, their yearly income approximated that earned through domestic farm production. For example, at the going rate in 1915 of $5 per birth, Mary Gerrard's midwifery income for 28 births would have equaled about $140 a year. This was less than the $175 one farm woman made from her eggs and chickens in a study from 1928–1930.[37]

The link between midwifery and women's traditional domestic roles was particularly clear in the case of Elin Nystrum, who practiced in Price County in 1910. Emigrating from Norway in 1905, Mrs. Nystrum, her husband, the Reverend John Nystrum, and their two young children settled first around Cambridge, Minnesota. While in Minnesota, Mrs. Nystrum studied midwifery for thirteen months with a local physician. By 1910, the family had moved again, this time to Ogema, in Price County. In 1911, she applied for a midwifery license from the state. The details of her license, together with evidence from the census and the birth certificates she filed, suggest that Mrs. Rev. John Nystrum (as she called herself) practiced midwifery for very traditional reasons.[38]

The lot of a minister's family was not an easy one in the nineteenth century, and the life of an immigrant minister's family was surely even more difficult. The family depended entirely on the support of parishioners, and this support varied according to the parishioners' own fortunes. One recent study, for example, points out that while in good years a minister's family could enjoy the modest comforts of the middle class, in bad years, the family might exist for months at a time on only apples and rice.[39] A minister's wife, then, had to know the tricks of frugal housekeeping.

While Elin Nystrum might conceivably have taken up midwifery in an attempt to supplement the family income, it is more probable that she learned midwifery as part of a traditional conception of the wifely duties of a minister. As the Reverend's wife, Nystrum enjoyed a high social position that carried a great deal of respect in her community. In addition to her own duties at home, ministers' wives were expected to help their husbands in the effort to save souls. In frontier areas, minister's wives had traditionally been exhorted to offer material healing and comfort in conjunction with their husbands' spiritual gifts, and the details of her practice suggest that Nystrum saw midwifery within this context. In 1910, she attended only two births, both within her own village. She was not found again in the birth records of the county.[40]

This domestic model of midwifery helps to explain some of the geographic limitations on midwifery practice. Rural women helped their neighbors, and midwives, trained or not, limited their practice in conformance with this domestic ideal. But rural neighborhoods in the late nineteenth and early twentieth centuries were often defined by immigrant groups as much as by geographic locations. Thus, an analysis of midwifery practice must also examine the strength of ethnic ties between midwives and birthing mothers.

Though both historians and contemporary analyses of midwives at the turn of the twentieth century have emphasized the link between immigrant midwifery practice and America's large cities, many immigrant midwives also moved to the rural midwest. Indeed, in the Children's Bureau study of Marathon County, Wisconsin, the authors remarked on the strong link between the practice of midwifery and the county's high percentage of European immigrants. Half of the midwives they found were "Polish women practicing in Polish settlements"; the rest were almost all German. In general, these midwives attended women of their own ethnic background, though one

German midwife reported that she had delivered the babies of a few native-born American families.[41]

As in Marathon County, midwives in Trempealeau, Price, and rural Dane County were almost all European immigrants. In these three rural counties, 40 of 88 midwives were from Scandinavia, usually Norway. The German-born numbered 16, and 19 were American-born, almost all the daughters of immigrant families.[42] Unlike the Marathon County midwives, however, these midwives did not always share the same ethnic background as their patients. But the differences between the counties illustrate the historical changes at work within the larger social context in which midwives practiced.

Price County, like Marathon County, was settled by European immigrant groups who came to this country in the years after the Civil War. Settling on the rough, uncleared land, the communities had very homogeneous ethnic populations. As in Marathon County, many communities were segregated by ethnic group and were described as "strongly foreign."[43] Midwifery practice showed the effects of this ethnic homogeneity. The patient population of thirteen Scandinavian midwives was 82 percent Scandinavian, and that of four German midwives was 71 percent German. The practice of even the American-born midwives showed this pattern: 92 percent of their patients had been born in this country.[44]

Eva Pasanen was representative of many midwives in Price County. Born in Finland, she was one of five Finnish midwives living in the largely Finnish township of Knox.[45] Delivering a total of eighteen babies in three sampled years (1910, 1915, and 1920), Pasanen was the most active of these five midwives. Despite the competition from other midwives in her community, however, the geographic location and ethnic background of her patients showed that the practice of midwifery had very tight cultural constraints. Like the other five Finnish midwives, all of Eva Pasanen's patients were Finnish. Furthermore, seventeen of her eighteen patients were from the small village of Brantwood.[46]

Eva Pasanen's midwifery practice reflected the relative youthfulness of the immigrant settlements in Price County. In Trempealeau and Dane County, however, most of the midwives were also European immigrants, but they did not exclusively attend families of their same ethnic backgrounds. For example, the ten Scandinavian midwives in

Trempealeau County had an average of 51 percent Scandinavian patients, while the eight Scandinavian midwives in Dane County had an average of only 41 percent Scandinavian patients.

The lower percentages of homogeneous practices in Trempealeau and Dane County can be explained in part by the rising number of American-born mothers who employed Scandinavian midwives. As the American-born children of immigrants had children of their own, they turned to the familiar birth attendant in the community. Indeed, as Sherbon and Moore found for the Polish community in Marathon County, this generation sometimes was more likely even than their mothers to hire midwives.[47] In 1890, for example, over 90 percent of the patients of Scandinavian midwives were also Scandinavian-born. By 1915, however, Scandinavian patients comprised only about 50 percent of a Scandinavian midwife's practice.

Yet not all American-born mothers sought out midwives from the old country. Over the years I examined, eleven midwives in Trempealeau and Dane counties were American-born, as were over 67 percent of their patients. But though these midwives continued an occupation of their European mothers, their midwifery practices were even more constrained. While the Scandinavian midwives in these two counties delivered an average of almost eleven babies, the American-born midwives attended about six. Indeed in Dane County, the native-born midwives attended only one to three births.[48]

Though no group of rural midwives ever built very large practices, the very small size of the practice of the American midwives indicates that the occupation of midwifery in America would not transcend its domestic roots. Unlike the foreign-born midwives, only one of these eleven American-born midwives, Elizabeth Briggs of Trempealeau County, applied for a state midwifery license.[49] Thus, instead of building a recognized occupation and identity for midwifery, these native-born midwives hearkened back to midwifery's most traditional model, that of the neighbor woman. Indeed, though Elizabeth Briggs may have regarded herself as a midwife, she had attended only fifty births in the thirty years she had been in practice.[50]

When Martha Ballard, a midwife in Augusta, Maine, died in 1812, she had delivered at least 998 births in thirty-five years of practice. A midwife summoned by families widely dispersed around her farming village, Ballard found herself by the early nineteenth century losing some patients to the young physicians who were eager to take even normal obstetrical cases.[51] This process of change in birth attendants proceeded throughout much the nineteenth century, and though more affluent urban women were the first to hire physicians, by the middle third of the nineteenth century, rural farm women increasingly asked for a physician to attend them.[52] Thus, by 1870 among the American-born farm families in Trempealeau and Dane Counties, there were no midwives like Martha Ballard. As in the Nanticoke Valley of upstate New York, native-born women who wanted a female birth attendant called in a relative or a next-door neighbor.

However, in the last half of the nineteenth century the native-born settlers of these rich agricultural areas were joined, indeed overwhelmed, by large numbers of European settlers. As the men brought their own farming methods, their wives brought a long tradition of midwifery. Settling in small, homogeneous communities, both sexes continued to practice their traditional crafts. However, as their sons and daughters intermingled with Americans, many ideas changed. Even European hospital-trained midwives went out only for their neighbors, and as they grew old and retired, few of their American-born daughters replaced them. This should not be surprising. There were few places to obtain training, and many second-generation immigrant mothers were emulating the native-born families of their communities and were hiring physicians to assist at their birthings. For rural midwives, midwifery had always been part of a strategy of neighborliness, and if the neighbors did not need you, then why go?

By contrast, the city offered urban midwives the possibility of building a large, even full-time practice. However, as the next chapter will show, even as some urban midwives adopted an entrepreneurial attitude in attracting patients, midwifery even within an urban context did not adopt a professional identity.

CHAPTER FOUR

Midwife Entrepreneurs
in the City

In 1884, Mary Gerrard, her husband, and their five children moved
from their farm at St. Joseph's Ridge into the nearby city of La-
Crosse, Wisconsin. Mrs. Gerrard, whose children ranged in age from
nine-year-old Nicolas to one-year-old Barbara, was pregnant with
what would be her sixth of seven children. But despite her increasing
family responsibilities, Mrs. Gerrard was a practicing midwife. Born
in Luxembourg in 1850, she had emigrated to the United States in
1872, and in 1874 she married a fellow countryman, Michael Gerrard.
Four years after her marriage, with three young children at home,
Mrs. Gerrard attended a three-month course at the Northwestern
Academy of Midwifery in Chicago, where she received a diploma in
1878.[1]

Like many families in the late nineteenth century, immigrant or
native-born, Mary Gerrard's family sought economic prosperity in
America's urban places. For Michael Gerrard, LaCrosse offered the
chance to make more money as a stonemason than he might as a
farmer. That the family prospered is shown by the fact that they
owned their home free and clear by 1905. The family home, in fact,
seemed crucial to the Gerrard children, who drifted in and out even
as adults.[2] But the family's security was not built solely by Michael.
Midwifery, it appeared, provided steadier work than that offered to
male artisans. In 1900, for example, he was unemployed for twelve
months, and Mary's midwifery practice was likely the family's sole
means of support. In fact, by 1905, Mary was listed as the head of
household.[3] Though her thirty-year-old son Nicolas was also living at

home, he had been employed as a painter the previous year for only seven months, while Mary had worked for the entire year.[4]

As Figure 4.1 shows, Mary Gerrard undoubtedly worked full-time as a midwife in the years after her family moved to LaCrosse. This was a dramatic change from the way she had practiced midwifery in St. Joseph's Ridge. There, constrained by both her rural locale and perhaps by her own growing family, Gerrard's practice in these years resembled the midwifery practice of many rural Wisconsin midwives. In 1878, for example, she delivered 16 babies, and in 1883, she delivered 25.[5] But once she began attending births in LaCrosse, the size of her practice increased markedly: from 45 births in 1885 to 134 in 1889, an almost sixfold increase over the average number of births she attended in St. Joseph's Ridge. With some minor dips in 1890 and 1891, her practice expanded to a high of 202 births in 1894. For several years during the middle of the 1890s, Mrs. Gerrard continued to attend almost 200 births per year, but by 1898, the number had begun to decline to an average of about 150 births per year. With some exceptions, she would keep up this pace until 1911, when the

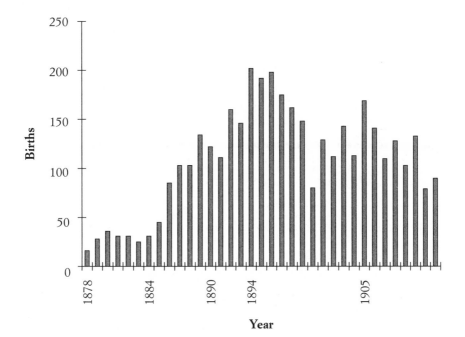

Figure 4.1 Mary Gerrard's midwifery practice, 1878–1912

total dipped to 79. In 1912, the last full year of her practice, she attended 90 births.[6]

Mary Gerrard's story demonstrates the point that above all, midwifery was a domestic craft for married women. Clearly, some women pursued it more intently than others. Even in the city, there were many midwives who continued to practice like those in rural Wisconsin. Of the 446 midwives identified in the two cities of Madison and Milwaukee, the majority, 354, were classified as less active. They delivered, on average, fewer than one baby per month, and most of the midwives in this group did not practice midwifery for more than a few years.

However, like Mary Gerrard, some urban midwives in Madison and Milwaukee in the late nineteenth century worked full-time at their craft. About 20 percent (92) of these urban midwives attended four or more births per month when they practiced midwifery, and unlike the less active urban midwives, these active practitioners also continued to practice over a number of years. Yet, in the end, though some of these busy women would deliver more babies per month than even most obstetricians, they did not advance a professional model for their craft. No matter how many babies they delivered, the practices of urban midwives were not structurally different from the very circumscribed neighborhood practices of rural midwives. Though city life offered some female birth attendants an opportunity to become midwifery entrepreneurs, these entrepreneurs never moved beyond the building of a large practice to the creation of an association that would make midwifery a permanent, professional occupation. Indeed, by the turn of the twentieth century, the number of midwives as active as Mary Gerrard had declined, and by 1920, no urban midwives, even those in Milwaukee, had large practices.[7]

Midwives as Entrepreneurs—The Active Urban Midwives

Eighty-eight Milwaukee midwives and four Madison midwives attended forty or more births in the sampled years between 1870 and 1920, which means that each midwife attended four or more births per month, as Table 4.1 demonstrates.

These practitioners must have been the most public and visible midwives, for though their numbers were small, they cared for the

70

Table 4.1   Active urban midwives: Number per year and number of deliveries

Year	No. of midwives	Mean no. of deliveries	
		Per month	Per year
1873	12	5.38	64.56
1877	19	5.88	70.56
1880	31	5.87	70.46*
1885	42	7.02	84.18*
1890	52	5.96	71.51*
1895	60	5.96	71.56*
1900	57	4.15	49.76*
1905	49	3.74	44.88
1910	38	4.57	54.82*
1915	33	4.34	52.08
1920	19	4.74	56.88

Sources: Sampled Birth Records, Milwaukee County, 1873–1920, Vital Records Office, Wisconsin Department of Health and Human Services, Madison, Wisconsin (WDHHS); Dane County, 1880–1910, Dane County Vital Records Office (DCVRO).

Notes: Madison midwives' births included in asterisked years only.

For both cities, active midwives were those who delivered more than forty total births over the course of the sampled birth records. For Milwaukee, the twelve-month totals were derived from a projection of the sampled three- or four-month totals for each year, but for Madison, the actual totals were used.

overwhelming majority of midwife-attended births. In Milwaukee, they constituted only 20 percent of the total number of midwives, and yet they delivered over 64 percent of the midwife-attended births. In Madison, the four active midwives (out of a total of thirteen) attended over 86 percent of the births where a midwife was present.[8] These active midwives also stayed visible by remaining in practice for extended periods of time. As a group, the eighty-eight Milwaukee midwives could be found in the records for an average of almost twenty years, while the Madison midwives averaged about twelve years.[9]

This level of activity and commitment indicated that these women viewed their midwifery practice as something more than giving occasional assistance to a neighbor in need. Also, unlike some rural neighbor women, these active urban practitioners sought training for their work. Indeed, of the seventy-three active midwives whose training could be determined, all were school-educated, the majority in Europe.[10]

Some active midwives were even busier than the averages shown in Table 4.1. Louisa Stange, a German-educated Milwaukee midwife, delivered twenty-one babies in February 1877. Figure 4.2, which details her work in that month, shows that Stange attended a birth 15 of the 26 days, and six times during the month she oversaw two births per day. Louisa Stange was one of the most active midwives in the birth sample: over the course of the twenty-one sampled months in the years between 1873 and 1890, she delivered 196 babies, an average of almost 10 babies per month. Emilie Roller, another active Milwaukee midwife, was even busier than Lousia Stange. Roller, who delivered the most children of any midwife in the study, attended 76 births within a three-month period in 1885. In fact, during June of 1885, she went to 21 childbirths over a twenty-nine day period.[11]

Attending more than a few births per month obviously disrupted a midwife's family life to some degree, and overseeing ten or more births per month on a regular basis made for what even modern nurse-midwives and obstetricians view as a full-time practice.[12] But despite these levels of activity, the family circumstances of midwives like Stange and Roller did not differ from those of other midwives. Neither were these practitioners elderly women who could do little else to

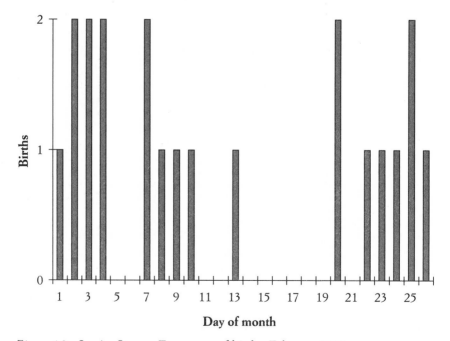

Figure 4.2 Louisa Stange: Frequency of births, February 1877

make money. Instead, for Mary Gerrard, Emilie Roller, and Louise Stange, midwifery was an occupation pursued during their middle-aged, not their elderly, years. Indeed, what is so striking about Emilie Roller's very busy midwife practice is that she was most active when she was relatively young and had school-aged children at home. In 1885, for example, her busiest year of those sampled, when she delivered 76 babies in a three-month period, she was thirty-nine years old and her two children were aged eleven and nine.

Typically, active midwives attended many deliveries during their forties and fifties and cut back on the pace of their practice as they approached their sixtieth birthday. Emilie Roller reduced the pace of her practice even by the time she reached her fifties. Figure 4.3, which gives Roller's three-month totals for every five years between 1880 and 1910, shows a distinct drop in the number of deliveries after 1895. By 1900, when she was fifty-four years old, she attended only 22 deliveries in a three-month period, and in 1910, at age sixty-four, she oversaw only 7 births between May 1 and July 31. Louisa Stange kept

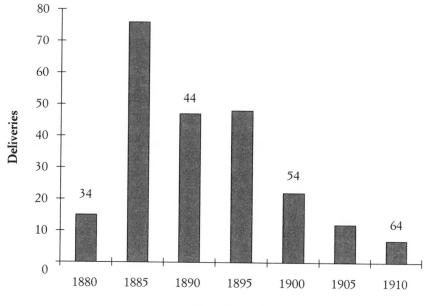

Figure 4.3 Emilie Roller: Three-month total deliveries (numbers over columns indicate Roller's age that year)

73

up the pace of her practice a little longer. Aged fifty-two in 1873, Stange delivered 49 children during February, March, and April. By 1880, when she was fifty-nine years old, her pace dropped to 34 births in three months. Stange continued a much lighter pace of practice as she grew older. Aged sixty-nine in 1890, she attended only 9 births between May and July.[13]

The relationship between Roller's and Stange's ages and the pace and the size of their practices was typical for all of Milwaukee's most active midwives, regardless of the years they delivered babies. Over the fifty years of this study, whether they started practice in 1877 or 1905,[14] most of these practitioners began to deliver babies when they were about thirty-nine years old, when they had an average of three children still at home. The first year, they attended an average of 42 births. Their practice continued to grow for eight to ten years, so that by their late forties when their pace of practice was at its peak, characteristically active midwives were delivering about 84 babies a year. As a female birth attendant reached her fifties, she began to take on fewer cases, and many active urban midwives ended their careers early in their sixties, when they might attend about 39 births.[15]

By attending school and by building a long-term, active practice, these urban midwives seemed to take a view of their work that went beyond that held by the neighbor-woman midwives. Certainly, the income of these active urban birth attendants was steadier and more substantial than the few dollars earned by a midwife who attended only a few births a year. Though evidence about the amount of money earned by midwives is fragmentary, some contemporary studies of midwives in various states and cities give rough approximations of the income produced by attending childbirths. Urban midwives, particularly those in large, industrial cities, earned more per delivery than rural midwives. For example, by the first decade of the twentieth century, midwives in East Boston, Massachusetts, and in Providence, Rhode Island, were reportedly paid about $15 per birth.[16] Detroit midwives charged an average of $10, but some female attendants accepted as little as $5.[17] Midwives in smaller urban areas, however, were paid much less. In Johnstown, Pennsylvania, for example, midwives charged between $3 and $5 for a delivery, and they would wait for payments or accept installment payments.[18]

Few midwife journals or diaries are still extant, and thus the completeness of Mary Gerrard's birth log allows us a rare chance to analyze an active, even entrepreneurial, midwife's income on a yearly and even case-by-case basis. Indeed, her careful notations in her birth log show that, for some women, midwifery could be financially worthwhile. Furthermore, her birth log demonstrates that Mary Gerrard only began to make significant sums of money when she moved to the relative urbanity of LaCrosse.[19]

During the six years that she and her family lived in St. Joseph's Ridge, Mrs. Gerrard's average income from her midwifery practice was $82.50. Her usual charge was $3.00, but her fees fluctuated several times each year, from nothing to as high as $5.00. With the move to LaCrosse in 1884, however, her individual fees as well as her yearly income from her midwifery practice rose sharply. Indeed, in the first year of practice in LaCrosse, her average fee had risen from $2.94 to $4.00, and by 1890, her average fee for a birth was $4.98. Though she continued to deliver a few babies for free, within four years of practice in LaCrosse, Mrs. Gerrard was charging a few patients as high as $10.00 for her attendance. Her yearly income reflected these higher charges and the rapid escalation of the pace of her practice. As Figure 4.4 shows, within three years of living in LaCrosse, her yearly income had more than quadrupled from her years in the country. By 1886 she was earning $341.50, and by 1890 her income was over $600. By 1896, she earned the most money in one year that she would ever make—$941 from attending 198 births. In the years following, her income began to decline slowly as the number of cases she attended also fell. By raising her rates per birth by the early twentieth century, however, Mrs. Gerrard made up part of this loss. In 1905, her average was $4.90 per birth. But in 1906, she had increased this to $6.65, and in 1908, her average had risen to $6.80. By 1912, her last full year in practice, she attended 90 births, at an average charge of $7.53, earning a total of $678.[20]

Though there are no records like Mary Gerrard's for midwives who practiced in the cities of Madison or Milwaukee, we can assume that midwives who practiced in these larger cities charged at least as much as she did. Thus midwives with very active practices like Mary Gerrard's stood a chance of making an income that would be noteworthy

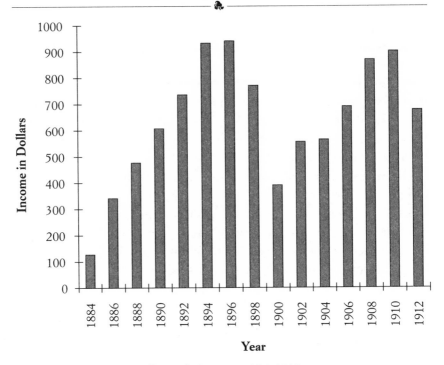

Figure 4.4   Mary Gerrard's yearly income, 1884–1912

among immigrant, working-class married women. Indeed, a full-time midwife might earn more money than women who worked for wages. While many women who worked in factories after 1900 were paid $6 to $8 per week, Mary Gerrard was earning from $12 to as much as $18 per week, an income achieved by few women in this period. Indeed, skilled men might expect to earn only $15 to $20 per week. Some years, in fact, her income was close to that of the average physician. While studies of physician incomes from the early years of the twentieth century indicate that they ranged from $1,000 to $1,500, a 1901 study pegged the average city doctor's income at only $730.[21]

Despite the impressive income levels achieved by these active, urban female birth attendants, they did not attempt to use their full-time status to promote a professional identity for midwifery. Like the rural midwives, the active urban midwives kept their practices based in their own neighborhoods. Thus, no matter how many patients a midwife attended in a year, her practice did not transcend the boundaries of a community defined by close ethnic and geographical ties.

The Geography of Practice of Urban Midwives

Anna Sampson, a midwife who practiced in rural Dane County in the last two decades of the nineteenth century, traveled at least three times to Madison to attend a birth. Her long journey, over twenty miles one way, was unusual not only for rural midwives, but also for those midwives who practiced in urban areas of Wisconsin. Indeed, of the entire group of midwives whose practices could be identified through birth certificates, Anna Sampson was the only midwife to travel such a long distance to attend a birth.[22]

Even within urban areas, where transportation was not a major hindrance, the geographic distances between urban midwives' homes and the location of their patients illustrates the essential neighborliness of midwifery practice. Midwives in Milwaukee or in Madison, regardless of the size of their practice, their years of experience, or their family circumstances, all delivered babies within specific areas close to their own homes.[23]

The continuing neighborliness of midwifery practice even in an industrialized, urban setting forces us to consider the relationship between gender and culture and the concept of professionalism in the early twentieth century. In terms of training, midwives who practiced in the cities I studied were different from those living in the rural areas. As noted in Chapter 1, it was not uncommon to find untrained neighbor women practicing as midwives in rural Wisconsin. In the state's urban areas, on the other hand, most midwives had sought some instruction, a move that might be interpreted as a step towards professionalization. By seeking some training, midwives in Milwaukee and Madison might have viewed their work as something beyond one neighbor helping another.

The evidence from an analysis of urban midwives' places of practice, however, demonstrates that rationalizing midwifery training did not lead to a wholly new conceptualization of midwifery. Consequently, even the active, full-time, urban midwives should be compared not to other health professionals in this period, but instead to the immigrant entrepreneurs who opened shops and started services within the immigrant community.

The story of Caroline Jaeger, the most active midwife in Madison, helps to illustrate this point. Born in Germany in 1855, Jaeger emigrated to the United States in 1881 with her husband Christian and at least one small child.[24] In July 1885, she graduated from the Milwaukee School of Midwifery and promptly registered with the Milwaukee Health Department. But Jaeger delivered very few babies in Milwaukee. Only a year later, in 1886, the family moved to Madison, where Christian Jaeger had found a job working for a local brewery.[25] The family's move to Madison, where midwives were less numerous, seems to have allowed Caroline to establish an active midwifery practice: in 1890, she attended thirty-two deliveries; and in 1895, she oversaw eighty-eight births.[26] Part of her success was undoubtedly related to her entrepreneurial efforts: she advertised her midwifery services in the *Madison City Directory* almost every year. These efforts obviously helped her to attract the notice of many parturient women, for Jaeger noted on her state midwifery license application in 1909 that she had attended at least 1,800 births.[27] Jaeger continued to deliver babies in Madison and to advertise in the city directory until 1914. By 1915, at the age of sixty, Jaeger retired from midwifery practice. Though Jaeger and her husband continued to live in Madison until at least 1919, she was not one of the few midwives delivering babies in the city in 1920.[28]

Though Caroline Jaeger built a very busy practice, her patients largely came from her own community. She and her husband lived in a section of the city largely populated by skilled and unskilled laborers, and 75 percent of her patients shared this class background. Furthermore, Jaeger did not seem to travel very far for a case: of 216 sampled births, only 2 were outside of Madison, and each of these births took place in rural towns just outside the city.[29] Madison midwives, as a rule, left the practice of midwifery in rural Dane county to local midwives.

Like Madison midwives, female birth attendants in Milwaukee also limited their the geographic reach of their practice. Midwives who lived in wards close to the edge of the city occasionally delivered babies in the towns bordering Milwaukee, but most of the city's midwives confined their practices to narrowly defined neighborhoods within the city. Sophia Bauersfeld, who lived in the eighth ward on Milwaukee's south side, for example, attended thirty-three births within a four-month period in 1873. She delivered twenty-four women who lived in her own eighth ward, seven mothers who lived in the adjacent fifth ward, and two who lived in the contiguous eleventh ward. Thus, all of the parturient women she delivered lived either in the same ward or in the two wards contiguous to hers (see Milwaukee ward maps, Figures 4.5, 4.6, and 4.7). Bauersfeld, an active midwife, never crossed into Milwaukee's north or east side neighborhoods. Margaret Fischer, who lived in Milwaukee's ninth ward in 1900, also delivered babies mainly in or near her neighborhood. About 31 percent of the births she attended occurred in the ninth ward, 20 percent were in the adjacent fifteenth ward, 27 percent were in the contiguous nineteenth ward, and 12 percent in the adjacent tenth and second wards. Only a very small percentage of Fischer's

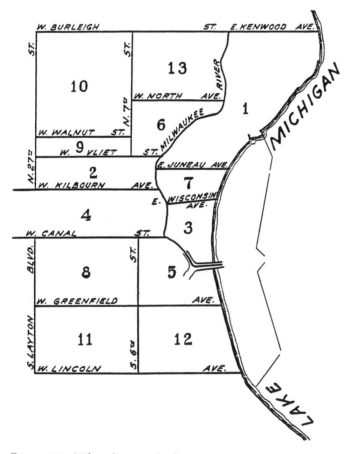

Figure 4.5 Milwaukee wards about 1873 (courtesy Manuscript Map Collection, Wisconsin State Historical Society)

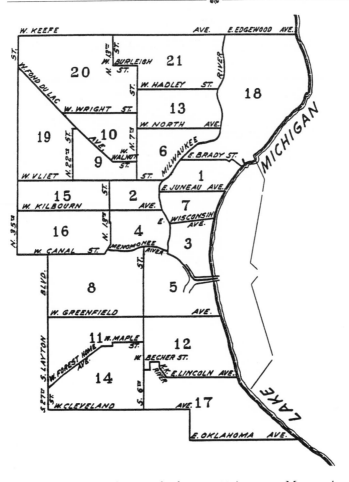

Figure 4.6 Milwaukee wards about 1900 (courtesy Manuscript Map Collection, Wisconsin State Historical Society)

births took her beyond her immediate neighborhood. The situation had not changed by 1920. Frances Jahnz, for example, was an active practitioner who lived in Milwaukee's twenty-fourth ward in 1920. Almost half of the births she attended came from her own ward (47 percent). Another 21 percent of her cases came from the adjacent eleventh ward, 16 percent from the fourteenth ward, and 9 percent from the eighth ward. She delivered a few babies in wards that were farther away, but still on the nearby south side. Pasqua Cafalu, who attended many of Milwaukee's Italian women, restricted her practice

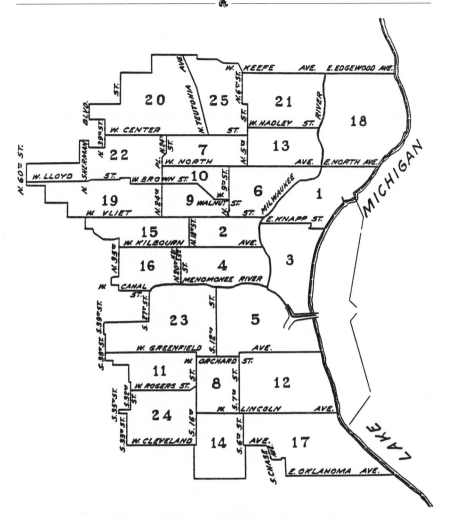

Figure 4.7   Milwaukee wards about 1920 (courtesy Manuscript Map Collection, Wisconsin State Historical Society)

even more than Jahnz. Cafalu, who lived in the third ward, delivered 87 percent of her patients in her own ward.[30]

The neighborly geographic confines of the midwife practices of Jahnz and Cafalu were typical of Milwaukee's urban female birth attendants. To test in a more rigorous way the relationship between a midwife's residence and the location of her patients, I constructed a mathematical index to measure the range of each attendant's practice.

For the years 1873, 1900, and 1920, the home ward of midwives with active practices was correlated with the wards where they attended births. For each midwife, a locality index was computed based on the distance of the ward of each birth from her home ward. Thus an index of zero would mean a practice based solely in the midwife's home ward, an index of one would mean a practice based largely in contiguous wards, and so on. For each of the three years, a mean index was then computed for all of the active midwives practicing that year.[31]

Though there were significant variations in the indices of individual midwives, the mean locality index for each of the three years never exceeded 1.000. That this index remained less than one shows that most midwives in this period attended births primarily within the neighborhood defined by their own ward. For midwives who practiced beyond their own ward, the south and the north sides of Milwaukee defined two larger, almost impermeable, neighborhoods. Thus, midwives living on the north side only delivered babies on north side wards, and midwives living on the south side never crossed the Menomonee River from the south Milwaukee wards.

The mean index for each of the three years did vary, however. For the active midwives practicing in Milwaukee in 1873, the index was 0.550, with a range of 0.200 to 0.950. In 1900, the mean index had risen somewhat, to 0.953. Some midwives, it seemed, were attending births further from home. That year, though twenty midwives had indices less than one, nineteen had locality indices greater than one, and one, Joanna Graf, had an index that approached 2.0. Graf was a German school-educated midwife who lived in the ninth ward. Unlike many midwives, her practice often took her beyond her own ward. For example, of the fourteen babies she delivered in three months in 1900, twelve were from wards other than her own. However, though her practice ranged more widely than that of many midwives, her practice was still confined only to the northwest wards of the city.[32]

Joanna Graf's midwifery practice in 1900, which included families from five different wards, was unusual. Anna Bernaski's midwifery practice, by contrast, was more predictive of the practice patterns of early twentieth-century midwives. With an index of 0.192, her practice was confined almost entirely to her own ward. Indeed, an analysis by street address showed that many of her patients were even more local. Of her 89 sampled deliveries between 1890 and 1905, 24 were from mothers who lived on her own street.[33]

Mrs. Bernaski's geographically very limited practice showed that the concept of midwifery as a neighborly occupation remained intact even in the beginning of the twentieth century. Though the mean locality index had risen somewhat by 1900, the increase was small, and not sustained: by 1920, the mean locality index had fallen to 0.777 for the nineteen active midwives still in practice.

The strong correlation between midwives' ethnicity and that of their patients are the best explanation for these female birth attendants' persistently small index of geographic diversity of practice. Throughout the period of this study, the northwest wards of Milwaukee were overwhelmingly German; Polish immigrants lived in two small areas of the north side and in the wards on the south side.[34] The small Italian community lived almost entirely in the third ward. Milwaukee's active midwives were drawn from all the immigrant communities within the city, and their patients almost always came from these same neighborhoods. This close congruence between the ethnic backgrounds of midwives and their patients did not change over time, and it is a key element in explaining the eventual decline of midwife practice.

With a mean index of 0.55, active midwives in 1873 stayed close to home. Home, in this case, meant the heavily German-speaking wards of Milwaukee, which comprised 32 percent of the city's population. Though there were large numbers of American-born and Irish immigrants living in the city, all of the active midwives were German-born, as were over 70 percent of their patients.[35] These midwives did attend a few American-born mothers, but judging from the neighborhood where they lived, these few were probably second-generation Germans.

By 1900, the number of midwives in the city had increased dramatically, as noted earlier. Of the fifty-six active midwives, there were nine Polish midwives in addition to the thirty-five German ones. Two midwives in this group were American-born second-generation Germans, and two others came from other European countries. As in 1873, the German-born midwives attended mostly German-born mothers (61.4 percent of their patients). A few other European immigrant groups (5.8 percent of their practice) consulted these

German midwives, but though some Polish immigrants came from German-speaking areas of Poland, only 1.1 percent of the practice of German midwives were Polish mothers.[36] Polish midwives, on the other hand, seemed to have more interaction with the German community. Almost half of their patients were listed as being German (46 percent), while 49 percent were Polish. This seeming interaction between ethnic groups was illusory, however. Most of the "German" patients lived in wards that were largely known to house immigrants from the German-speaking areas of Poland, and their identification as "German-born" did not reflect their actual heritage.[37]

By 1920, though the active midwives in the sample continued to have neighborhood-based, ethnic practices, the significant decline in the number of foreign-born families in Milwaukee would exact a large toll on the practice of midwifery. Active urban midwives had always relied on large numbers of immigrant women, but the percentage of foreign-born in Milwaukee fell from over 45 percent in 1900 to about 24 percent in 1920.[38] As Figure 4.8 indicates, these dates correspond to declines in midwifery practice in the city. After 1895, as the number

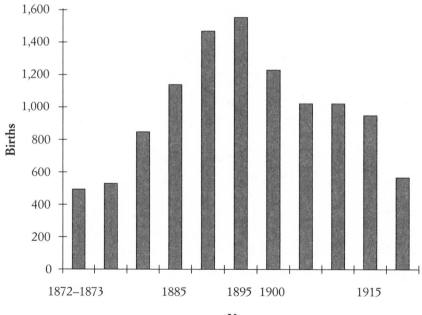

Figure 4.8 Births attended by Milwaukee midwives, by year

84

of births attended by all midwives decreased, the number of births attended by each midwife also fell.

The dwindling percentages of same-ethnic-group patients between 1900 and 1920 are key to explaining the declining numbers of midwives and the decrease in the number of midwife-attended births in this period. All but one of the midwives in 1920 were born in Europe, and, as had been the case in the past, many of their patients were members of the same ethnic group. But many midwives had increasing numbers of American-born mothers, the second generation of many immigrant neighborhoods.[39] In fact, with two exceptions, the size of the practice for each ethnic group of Milwaukee midwives in 1920 could be predicted by the percentage of fellow countrywomen that they attended. Thus it was not surprising that Pasqua Cafalu, an Italian-born midwife who attended only Italian mothers, delivered 31 babies in a three-month period. For the seven active Polish midwives in 1920, the three-month mean was 17.1 deliveries. Polish patients made up about 54 percent of their practice, and the number of American-born mothers had risen from a negligible 1.5 percent in 1900 to almost 32 percent. The decline in European-born patients was most pronounced for the German midwives, and it helps to explain why they delivered an average of only 9.9 babies in a three-month period. Only 29.4 percent of their patients in 1920 were German-born, while almost 43 percent of their patients were American-born.[40]

The decline in the foreign-born population is also reflected in the decreasing number of active midwives after 1900. By arranging the active Milwaukee midwives into cohorts by the year they began their practice, Table 4.2 shows a substantial decrease in the number of active midwives by 1900. Indeed, of the eighty-eight active Milwaukee midwives, only eleven began their practice in the twentieth century, and all four of the active Madison midwives had begun their practice by 1890.[41]

The Decline of Midwifery

While ninety-two urban midwives had practices that distinguished them as very active, even entrepreneurial, female birth attendants, many more urban practitioners attended only a few births per year.

Table 4.2 Active Madison and Milwaukee midwives: Number by year starting practice

Cohort year	Number in cohort
1873	12
1877	9
1880	11*
1885	15*
1890	21*
1895	13
1900	6
1905	4
1910	1
1915	0
1920	0

Sources: Sampled Birth Records, Milwaukee County, 1873–1920, WDHHS; also Dane County, 1880–1910, DCVRO.
Note: Madison midwives' births included in asterisked years only.

But little distinguished these less active midwives from those with larger practices. Whether they delivered only a few or many babies, most urban midwives had been born in Europe (particularly Germany), were married to artisans, and had several children at home.[42] Furthermore, midwives of both Polish and German background could be found in either group.[43] Perhaps most important, however, many of the less active urban midwives demonstrated the same type of commitment to a midwifery career as those female birth attendants who had large practices. Thus, while many urban midwives, like their rural counterparts, undoubtedly kept their practices small because they viewed their work as merely helping out a neighbor or a female relative, other midwives with small practices showed that they wished to expand this limited vision of midwifery. Many of the less active attendants registered with the Milwaukee Board of Health, an indication that they considered themselves true midwives and wanted to be allowed to practice.[44] These women had also pursued training: 15 midwives with small practices had apprenticed themselves to Milwaukee doctors, and 122 of these less active practitioners had received school training, mostly in Milwaukee.[45]

The major difference between the group of midwives who attended large numbers of births and those who oversaw only a few had to do with when each group began its practice. By the twentieth century, as more urban midwives sought out training and registration regardless of their ethnic background, the size of their practices was 83 percent less than that of nineteenth-century midwives.[46] When the members of each group were cross-tabulated by their appearance in the census, the women who attended many deliveries turned out to be older women who were more likely to have first appeared in the early census years of 1870 and 1880 and less likely to have first appeared in the 1905 and the 1910 censuses.[47] The dates that midwives registered with the Milwaukee Health Department and the schools that the less active midwives attended showed the same historical effects. The mean date for the 77 active practitioners who could be traced to the Health Department Register was 1887, while the mean date for the 168 less active midwives who registered with the Health Department was 1893.[48] These younger midwives, like their older fellow immigrant midwives, demonstrated their commitment to school training. But unlike the older active female birth attendants, most of these midwives went to school in Milwaukee. Locally trained midwives had an average graduation date of 1880, while the average date for the foreign-trained practitioners was 1866, fourteen years earlier.[49]

Though each ethnic group of less active midwives had equally small numbers of patients, there were differences in the demographic characteristics of their practice. For the German midwives who began their practice early in the twentieth century, the community of women patients increasingly was comprised of second-generation, American-born German immigrants. Thus, while German patients made up almost 62 percent of the practice of active German midwives, German families comprised only 50 percent of the practice of the less active German midwives. Conversely, the percentage of American-born patients was significantly higher for the less active midwives (over 36 percent) than it was for the active group (over 27 percent of their practice).[50] For the Polish midwives, the number of Polish and Polish-German patients also declined, but there were considerable variations among the midwives, and no statistical significance could be shown. In fact, the percentage of American-born patients for each group remained steady, at about 12 percent of a typical practice.[51]

Clearly by the turn of the twentieth century, within the urban, ethnic communities of Madison and Milwaukee, younger female birth attendants were not building full-time practices as their counterparts did in the 1880s or even the 1890s. As Table 4.1 shows, the number of active midwives rapidly declined after 1900. By 1920, in fact, the number of active midwives, 19, was 66 percent less than it was in 1900. Furthermore, the mean number of births overseen by even the active midwives declined from a little over 7 per month in 1885 to about 4.5 by 1910. As Table 4.3 shows, this process of decline had begun in the last decades of the nineteenth century, and the less active midwives' percentage of total deliveries increased throughout the fifty-year sample period. Thus, in 1877, the less active group accounted for less than one-sixth of all midwife deliveries, but by 1915, they attended more than half of all midwife-attended births. To what do we account this decline in the number of midwives and the number of midwife-attended births?

Previous studies of late nineteenth-century midwives in the United States have usually focused on the legal status of midwives and the struggles of predominantly elite physicians to regulate midwifery. The resulting interpretation has portrayed midwives as victims of an all-powerful and sometimes sexist medical establishment. Midwives, according to this view, were poor, isolated practitioners who did not have the resources to stand up to their critics.[52] But this analysis has largely left midwives' own lives out of the story, and it begs the ques-

Table 4.3   Less active Milwaukee midwives: Number of midwives, number of deliveries, percent of total deliveries

Year	No. of midwives	No. of deliveries	Percent of all midwife deliveries
1872	6	39	29.8
1873	11	103	28.5
1877	15	81	15.3
1880	21	129	15.2
1885	61	279	24.5
1890	95	580	39.5
1895	114	533	34.3
1900	126	529	43.0
1905	107	473	46.2
1910	105	518	50.6
1915	87	519	54.7
1920	65	296	52.3

Source: Birth Records, Milwaukee County, 1872–1920, WDHHS.

tion of why midwives remained isolated practitioners and did not stand up to their critics.[53]

As this and previous chapters have shown, the practice of midwifery was tied to the gender and the shared ethnic backgrounds of midwives and their patients. These questions of gender and culture were in turn tied to defining the nature of the "professional" in early twentieth-century America. In the early 1900s Americans were increasingly celebrating the role of the professional, and childbirth was but one of many realms where questions were raised about the need for an expert. Indeed, as Judith Walzer Leavitt has pointed out, childbearing women, who were as aware as anyone about the manifold dangers of birth, helped to shape this process of change. As Leavitt and others have shown, as early as the first third of the nineteenth century, even the promise of the relief of suffering through the application of science was enough to convince many native-born white women to hire physicians.[54]

But while the role of the physician conveyed the idea of the scientific expert, the role of the midwife did not. Though the physician might be either male or female, midwives could only be women, and thus midwifery remained tied to culturally understood definitions about gender and knowledge. As Chapter 1 showed, even the establishment of midwifery schools did not confer a new "expert" status to women who sought out training. Furthermore, as Chapters 3 and 4 have shown, trained midwives did not behave differently from those who had a more casual understanding of the subject. Academically trained midwives might better understand the anatomy of the pelvis, and they might use new aseptic techniques for delivery, but the old relationship of female neighbor helping female neighbor did not change. Indeed, contemporary observers of midwives expressed surprise when they found that by the twentieth century few midwives continued to perform household tasks for the parturient woman.[55]

These issues, however, were mediated within a given community, whether immigrant or native-born; and, as the next few chapters show, the rise of the physician as birth attendant must also be considered within a cultural context.

CHAPTER FIVE

Educating Physicians

In his 1899 presidential address to the State Medical Society of Wisconsin, Dr. Herman Reineking pointed to what he saw as the most obvious reason for employing a physician birth attendant. "Is it not appalling to think," he insisted, "that woman, in the most perilous hours of her life, should be left to the tender mercies of uneducated and as a rule superstitious and dirty persons, instead of being assured the benefit of every means that science offers for her protection and the amelioration of her suffering?"[1] As Dr. Reineking explained, only a physician could offer this new science. "No one, except the educated physician, can ever give the parturient woman the aid, protection and amelioration of suffering to which she is entitled."[2]

Dr. Reineking's impassioned advocacy of the superiority of the educated, scientific physician was a popular theme in the medical literature in the late nineteenth and early twentieth centuries. Like Dr. Reineking, many physician-leaders argued that new scientific discoveries had provided them with the expert knowledge and the tools that were needed to solve the problems of disease and ill health. Midwives, they argued, lacked the education and, even more important, the appreciation of the fundamental knowledge of nature that the new scientific medical training instilled. In particular, obstetricians argued that childbirth was an inherently pathologic process that even many physicians were ill-equipped to monitor. Midwives, these specialists asserted, dragged down the standards of scientific medicine because the low level of their care diminished both physicians' and the public's expectations of what constituted good obstetrics. As one Illinois physician argued, childbirth was no place for an "ignorant woman" who "never can grasp the broad fact that the delivery of a woman is a serious problem." "Midwifery," he concluded, "is not in consonance with the spirit or intent of modern scientific medicine."[3]

Even as national medical leaders identified a "midwife problem" in the United States, the number of midwife-attended births began to fall. Statistics illustrate the steep decline: in 1904, almost 53 percent of Milwaukee's babies were delivered by midwives and 47 percent were overseen by physicians; statewide in that year, midwives attended about 35 percent of births and physicians about 63 percent.[4] By 1915, however, only 26 percent of babies in Milwaukee and 13 percent in the entire state were born with the aid of a midwife.[5] Wisconsin paralleled a national trend. In 1910, about half of all American babies were delivered by midwives. By 1930, only 15 percent of all births in the United States were midwife-attended,[6] though the figures differed for urban and rural areas. The public, it seemed, was listening to medicine's call for physician expertise in the birthing room.

But the rhetoric of the scientifically educated physician far outran the reality. Though science was investing physicians with new authority in the birthing room, this authority was gained more from the promise than from the actual pedagogical content of medical education. In this chapter I analyze the medical training of 912 licensed physicians who practiced in four Wisconsin counties between about 1870 and 1930. I describe the overall medical education of these 912 doctors, mostly general practitioners, focusing specifically on their obstetrical education.

While the opinions of national medical leaders about the deficiencies of the curricula of many late nineteenth-century medical schools have been well documented, little research has been done on the graduates of these schools, particularly the general practitioners who attended the typical, nonselect medical schools of the late nineteenth and early twentieth centuries. Yet these general practitioners were the ones who presided at the majority of physician-attended births. Thus, an analysis of these nonelite schools, and their state and local leaders, points to an understanding of how the Progressive Era public was convinced of the "legitimate complexity" of science and the need for institutionalized professional authority.[7]

Assessing Physician Education for Obstetrical Practice

Though most late nineteenth-century physicians saw many patients in the course of a general practice, not every doctor saw maternity patients. Thus, to assess the preparation for the practice of obstetrics, I analyzed the education of only those physicians who delivered babies in the course of their practice.[8] The large birth certificate sample from the four counties provided the names of 1,149 possible physicians. I was able to determine the educational backgrounds of 912 of these physicians from the data on the licenses filed by physicians who complied with the Wisconsin Medical Practice Act or from the "Directory of Milwaukee Physicians, 1834–1914," in Louis F. Frank's *The Medical History of Milwaukee, 1834–1914.*[9] To assess the class and ethnic backgrounds of these physicians, I linked 598 physicians to either the federal or the Wisconsin state census. As with the midwife census study, each physician was linked to the first census where he or she could be found, and demographic data about family structure, ethnic background, and other social factors were collected.[10] In order to study changes over time, the physicians were divided into two groups by the date that they registered for a license. This dividing date reflected an important new emphasis by Wisconsin's physician leaders on the importance of premedical education as preparation for medical school.

As historians have noted, the imposition of entrance requirements to medical schools lagged behind all other aspects of educational reform. Even at some of the better medical schools, applicants could gain admission without a high school diploma. In 1904, the American Medical Association's newly formed Council on Medical Education formulated minimum standards for medical education that included a premedical requirement of at least four years of high school.[11] Wisconsin responded to these standards by inserting a provision in the Medical Practice Act that required physicians who registered after 1906 to have the premedical education equivalent of a high school degree. Thus, the physicians included in the pre-1905 section make up an older group, many of whom were trained before the advent of significant educational reforms; most of the doctors in the post-1905 group had a significantly longer medical education. As this chapter illustrates, however, the call for a science-based education did not extend very far, and even physicians trained in the early decades of the twentieth century had very little understanding of what Dr. Reineking had termed the "means that science offers for [the childbearing woman's] protection and the amelioration of her suffering."[12]

Though by the end of the nineteenth century more women were entering medical school, the physician expertise in Wisconsin's birthing rooms was largely represented by men. The overwhelming majority of the 912 physicians in my sample were male (98.4 percent). Of the fifteen women physicians identified, ten registered before 1905. Six of the ten were educated at regular medical schools, and four had graduated from Chicago's homeopathic Hahnemann Medical College. All of the women physicians in the sample lived in either Milwaukee or Madison. Though it would have been interesting to compare the maternity practices of male and female physicians, the small number of women doctors in this sample precluded a comparative analysis. However, recent research comparing the practice of male and female physicians suggests that most women doctors saw themselves as full-fledged health professionals.[13] With women doctors making up less than 2 percent of the sample, the question of gender distinctions among practitioners reduces to the differences between midwives and physicians.

Medical Education before 1905

For most American doctors who sought a medical education between the end of the Civil War and approximately 1890, medical school was not a post-college degree program. Indeed, most medical students had little or no college preparation, and many had not graduated from high school. The medical school curriculum was minimal. The standard program consisted of two four-month lecture terms held in the winter months, with the second-term lectures merely repeating those of the first.[14] Students attended didactic lectures for all of the seven courses of the typical medical school curriculum; clinical courses, such as obstetrics, as well as basic sciences, such as anatomy, were taught as lectures. In addition, as late as 1880 only ten American medical schools had introduced a graded curriculum; as a result, students in most schools did not have to master preclinical subjects, such as anatomy, before they began learning surgery and obstetrics.[15]

By the early 1870s, several elite American medical schools had re-organized their schools' curricula and structure. Reformers, among them Charles Eliot of Harvard University and others at the University of Pennsylvania and the University of Michigan, assumed new authority and control of their medical schools. They increased their schools' terms from five months to six or nine months, imposed a graded curriculum, and lengthened the program from two to three years. By 1890, these schools had also introduced laboratory sciences into the medical curriculum, and they had begun to require that incoming students have at least a high school diploma and preferably several years of college preparation.[16]

The opening of The Johns Hopkins Medical School in 1893 set a new standard for American medical education. Basing its program on the model of the German medical schools, Johns Hopkins established "medical education as a field of graduate study, rooted in basic science and hospital medicine."[17] Establishing a four-year graded curriculum from the start, Hopkins also required a bachelor's degree from every matriculant. The real significance of this school, however, was that it joined science and research ever more firmly to clinical hospital practice. Students no longer just observed a clinical case in the vast confines of the school's amphitheater or by quickly walking the wards; at Johns Hopkins, they attended patients, observed their symptoms, and received hands-on experience in every clinical specialty.[18] For many national medical leaders and Progressive-Era reformers, The Johns Hopkins Medical School embodied the essence of the new scientific medicine.

Though Harvard, Johns Hopkins, and other, mostly northeastern medical schools offered a new model for medical education, most of the 604 Wisconsin physicians who registered with the state prior to 1905 had been trained in an older American educational paradigm that emphasized apprenticeships and didactic lectures. For most of these doctors, about a year of their education had involved working with a preceptor: 329 (70.3 percent of 468 known cases) indicated they had worked with a preceptor, 139 (29.7 percent of known) had not.[19] Furthermore, though 36 percent of Milwaukee's physicians in 1860 had trained in Germany, by the last decades of the nineteenth century, Wisconsin's doctors, including those in Milwaukee, were largely American-trained. Only 49 of the 604 physicians in the pre-

1905 group (7.9 percent) had graduated from foreign schools: 30 from German or Austrian medical schools, 7 from Norwegian or British schools, 8 from Canadian, and 4 from Polish.[20] Most of these physicians were older immigrant physicians: their mean date of graduation was 1881, compared with 1891 for the group as a whole and a mean date of 1892 for the American-trained physicians.[21] In addition, the wars over therapeutics that had so bitterly divided medical practitioners earlier in the nineteenth century were settled in Wisconsin in favor of the medical regulars. Of 520 pre-1905 registrants who identified a school of practice, 471 were "regulars," and only 49 were "sectarians." Of these 30 were homeopaths, 15 were "eclectic," and 4 had various affiliations.[22]

The vast majority of doctors in Wisconsin who began their practice before 1905 attended medical schools that were slow to adopt the reforms instituted in the elite schools in the 1880s and 1890s.[23] Most of the regular physicians took three or four courses of lectures (the mean was 3.52 years), and the few sectarian physicians (i.e., homeopaths or other "irregular" physicians) took only two or three courses, a significant difference that reflected the increasing problems faced by sectarian schools by the end of the nineteenth century.[24] Whether regular or sectarian, most Wisconsin physicians attended midwestern medical schools. In fact, about 65 percent of the sampled physicians who registered or began their practice prior to 1905 attended ten schools, as shown in Table 5.1.[25] Nine of these ten were in the Midwest, and the seven Milwaukee and Chicago schools graduated 353 of the 385 doctors (91.7 percent) who attended the ten schools. The Chicago schools were particularly popular, because though a large number of physicians were born in Wisconsin (at least 39 percent), residents of the state prior to 1894 who wished to obtain medical training were forced to go out of state.[26]

Rush Medical College, which graduated the largest percentage of Wisconsin doctors, was typical of the three popular regular schools in Chicago. Founded in 1843, Rush quickly became very large, and for some time during the nineteenth century it graduated the largest medical school classes in the United States. Like many proprietary medical schools of the late nineteenth century, Rush adopted educational reform slowly: it approved a two-year graded curriculum in the late 1870s and did not extend its course to three years until 1885.

Table 5.1 Wisconsin medical graduates, pre-1905: The ten most frequently attended medical schools (*n* = 385, total *n* = 604)

School	Location	No. of graduates	% of total
Rush	Chicago	107	17.7
Milwaukee Medical	Milwaukee	83	13.7
Wisconsin Physicians & Surgeons	Milwaukee	53	8.8
Chicago Physicians & Surgeons	Chicago	39	6.5
Northwestern	Chicago	36	6.0
Hahnemann	Chicago	24	4.0
University of Michigan	Michigan	12	2.0
Iowa Physicians & Surgeons	Iowa	11	1.8
Bennett	Chicago	11	1.8
New York Physicians & Surgeons	New York City	9	1.5

Sources: Louis Frederick Frank, "Directory of Milwaukee Physicians, 1834–1914," *The Medical History of Milwaukee, 1834–1914* (Milwaukee: Germania Publishing Co., 1915), pp. 238–271; also Board of Medical Examiners, Physician Licenses (Series 1606) and Register of Physicians (Series 1621), Archives Division, Wisconsin State Historical Society, Madison, Wisconsin.

In the early 1890s, Rush expanded its requirements for graduation to include four years of twenty-one week terms each year, but the school granted advanced standing to students with four years of college. At the same time that the school increased the length of the medical school program, it began to require more rigorous premedical training. By 1898, Rush mandated that potential students attend four years of high school; by 1904, two years of college were required.[27]

When the Wisconsin College of Physicians and Surgeons and the Milwaukee Medical College opened in Milwaukee in 1894, many Wisconsin medical students were able to matriculate closer to home than Chicago. Established by groups of local physicians as profit-making ventures, both Wisconsin medical colleges were slow to adopt the curricular changes adopted by even other midwestern schools. Neither school, for example, extended its training to a four-year program until 1900, and though high-school diplomas were required for admission, the Milwaukee Medical College was accused by the Milwaukee County Medical Society in 1902 of admitting students who lacked high school degrees.[28]

Even as many medical schools struggled to meet new standards of medical education at the end of the nineteenth century, obstetrics education lagged behind. Indeed, though the aura of science was investing physicians with new authority in the birthing room, many physicians in this period had significantly less education in obstetrics than school-educated midwives.[29]

In the late nineteenth and early twentieth centuries, many schools instructed students in obstetrics through a combination of lectures, recitations, practice on a manikin, and, in a few fortunate instances for their students, delivering poor women in their homes. For most students and teachers, this system was not altogether satisfactory. As George J. Engelmann wrote in 1888, "The student is taught the management of pathological cases, but how to guard his patient against their occurrence, the practical management of simple labor, examination, and manipulation, he must learn by experience."[30] Wisconsin doctors training before 1905, like their colleagues throughout the United States, learned obstetrics in this way.[31]

At the University of Michigan, for example, where twelve Wisconsin students received their training, though the school was considered by some to be the best school in the Midwest, the obstetrical training was limited mostly to a series of didactic lectures and demonstrations in an amphitheater. Though 382 hours of the curriculum was devoted to obstetrics and gynecology, most students spent the majority of their time two afternoons a week, three in the afternoon to six or seven o'clock in the evening, sitting "on the hard benches of the operating theater, high above the pit, where students could see nothing and understand little of what was occurring at the operating table."[32] Indeed, until 1900, Michigan graduates could begin their medical practice without ever having actually observed a delivery.

Most of the actual "clinical training" given to Michigan and other medical school students focused on the obstetrical manikin. Indeed, for many medical students who attended schools where there were no parturient women patients for hands-on clinical training, these manikins provided students with their sole experience with labor and delivery. In other schools, where lying-in patients were available but the number was limited, it was considered "advisable that the students be taught the rudiments of palpation, touch, and pelvimetry upon the manikin, so that they will know exactly what they are to do when they examine the patients in the wards, whereby clinical material is economized, and the patients saved considerable annoyance."[33]

Some medical schools and physician teachers established extensive obstetrical programs around the manikin. Dr. Eliza Root, an instructor at the Woman's Medical College of Northwestern University, detailed such a program in 1899. She suggested junior and senior courses in obstetrics for four-year schools and a junior course in normal obstetrics only for three-year programs. Her course required a comprehensive study of the pelvis and work in embryology before students would undertake extensive work on the manikin. This manikin work, Root maintained, would teach the student a great deal about birth:

> The drill on the manikin with the normal fetus, or with the dummy, is of supreme importance to the student. He sees and understands for himself the wonder-inspiring process of accommodation of the fetal diameters to the pelvic dimensions. He begins to accept as demonstrable truth what before seemed only half truth, and he is willing to again and again repeat his assigned task, for he is beginning to love the work, and to desire its mastery.[34]

When proficient in dealing with normal presentations, the student was then instructed in other vertex presentations, then on breech and other difficult deliveries. As Root outlined,

> During these different exercises on the manikin he should be taught the judicious use of the hands in aiding spontaneous delivery; . . . and the different manual methods of delivering the after-coming head . . . The student must not be passed too rapidly over the exercises on the manikin, or he becomes confused, and fails to divine important steps one from another. Mastering each step as he advances, he becomes more and more interested in the work.[35]

For the senior medical student, Root outlined a program of teaching "pathologic obstetrics." Students were taught operative obstetrics, particularly the use of forceps, again through drills on the manikin.

Learning correct use of the forceps was important. As Root explained, "No student should be allowed to leave his school without a safe knowledge of this instrument, which he will gain only by the study of it as a mechanical appliance, and by thorough drill in its use on the manikin."[36]

Root's program in obstetrical training relied heavily on the manikin, though she did urge that "practical work in obstetrics should be required of each student before graduation." However, she provided so few details about what a practical program should provide for the student that it is evident that her students saw few actual patients. Indeed, her final recommendation was that a student should gain clinical experience by taking "a post-graduate course in some good maternity, of value to him for further preparation for the practice of obstetrics."[37]

Though, as noted above, many of the 604 Wisconsin physicians had precepted with a senior physician, it is likely that few of them actually assisted their mentor doctor in his private obstetrical cases. As Charles Rosenberg has found, most physicians would not allow their student preceptors to attend the deliveries of their private patients. Thus, the only place a student physician might learn clinical obstetrics was in a hospital or through a home delivery service.[38]

But the possibilities for hospital experience were also quite limited. Like most post–Civil War American medical school graduates, the Wisconsin doctors had very little clinical experience in a hospital. Though the physicians in this group spent an average of 7.3 months in the hospital either before or after graduation, 271 of 475 (57.1 percent of the cases where hospital experience could be ascertained) never had any hospital experience.[39] This lack of training was typical of the average medical student's experience in this period, and it did not differ by the later urban or rural location of the physicians' practice.[40] Further training required money and family connections, something most Wisconsin physicians lacked.

To gain more clinical experience, some nineteenth-century physicians went on after medical school to attend a postgraduate course. Others went to Europe to train in the great German or Austrian hospitals or laboratories. However, many doctors could not afford these routes to further training. A few hospitals offered positions as "house pupils" to medical graduates who wished further clinical training, but as with the other routes, securing these scarce positions required that the applicant come from a socially prominent family.[41]

If physicians trained in the late nineteenth century had very little actual hospital experience for all their clinical subjects, hospital or outpatient obstetrical training was even more meager. At the University of Michigan, for example, a lucky student might see one of the ten or twelve obstetrical patients per year cared for at the university hospital. Even with the establishment of a small obstetrical hospital at Ann Arbor in 1903, students saw very few patients, as the ward had only thirty beds and parturient women remained hospitalized for many weeks postpartum.[42] By the turn of the twentieth century, a few other schools had instituted home deliveries by medical students. But the learning experience in this situation could be haphazard, as students were usually sent unaccompanied to attend the patients.[43]

Though home delivery instruction came under increasing fire from some educators early in the twentieth century, at least students were able to observe a birth at close range, and they even could perform the delivery themselves.[44] At many medical schools, however, most students never got to deliver a baby at all. Indeed, they were lucky when they could just observe a birth. For example, all students who attended Northwestern University Medical School between 1870 and 1891 witnessed a delivery only if they could bribe a woman to deliver her baby in the school's amphitheater. Ironically, the famous obstetrician Joseph B. DeLee, a graduate of Northwestern, later recalled that he had been fortunate to have watched two such deliveries during his student years.[45]

Students training at the Milwaukee schools had even less clinical experience than the pre-1905 group who trained in Chicago or at other schools. Both the Milwaukee Medical College and the Wisconsin College of Physicians and Surgeons were affiliated with small hospitals, whose patients were mostly surgical cases.[46] At the Milwaukee Medical College, the sixty-eight graduates by 1905 reported a mean of only 1.94 months of hospital experience, and almost 75 percent of them had no hospital time; the forty physicians who trained at the Wisconsin College of Physicians and Surgeons in the same time period reported a mean of 3.1 months, with 82 percent having no hospital time.[47] As late as 1910, clinical obstetrical experience at both Milwaukee schools was limited to amphitheater teaching only. Neither school had at-home delivery services for teaching medical students.[48]

In short, when they began their practice of medicine, many of Wisconsin's pre-1905 medical school graduates were lucky if they had even witnessed a birth. The clinical facilities at the Chicago and Milwaukee medical schools where most of these doctors trained were meager, so it was not surprising that many physicians later recalled their fear when, as young graduates, they were called to a delivery.[49]

Medical School Reform and Clinical Teaching after 1905

In his famous 1910 report to the Carnegie Foundation on the state of American medical education, Abraham Flexner indicted the quality of education offered by most American medical schools. He recommended that many medical schools make significant improvements in their laboratories, libraries, curricula, and clinical facilities. Many schools, he concluded, were beyond hope for improvement, and he urged them to close or merge with other schools. But, as a number of historians have pointed out, by 1910, despite the public furor over medicine inspired by Flexner's report, American medical education was actually the best it had ever been. Most schools had already begun reforming their entrance requirements and their curricula in the 1880s and 1890s, so that by 1893 over 90 percent of American medical schools had a three-year program. In addition, students were better prepared for medical school, and by 1900 even the weaker medical schools had instituted demanding courses and curricula.[50]

The credentials of the 308 Wisconsin physicians in the study who registered after 1905 shows that the effect of medical education reform in the first decades of the twentieth century had began to filter down to even the small, less elite schools of the Midwest. Similar to their earlier colleagues in terms of social backgrounds, the Wisconsin physicians who registered after 1905 were mostly native-born, and they continued to study close to home, attending most of the same medical schools as their predecessors. However, school training had replaced apprenticeships. Few doctors in the post-1905 group studied with preceptors: only 35 doctors (11.7 percent of known 298) had studied with a preceptor whereas 263 (88.3 percent) had not.[51] Also, unlike their older colleagues, these younger physicians studied at schools with four-year programs: 277 of 308 doctors in this sample (89.9 percent) graduated after four years of medical education; only 37 doctors (12.0 percent) had two or three years of medical school.[52] As with the earlier group, most of these schools were in the Midwest. As Table 5.2 demonstrates, 71.4 percent of doctors in this group (220 of 308) attended ten schools, all of them in Milwaukee or Chicago.

Even the few sectarian physicians in the post-1905 group were better educated than their older colleagues. The fourteen sectarians in this group had a mean of 3.57 years of medical lectures, significantly more than the pre-1905 sectarians, whose mean number of lectures was only 2.88.[53] However, this mean still lagged significantly behind the mean number of medical lectures attended by their regular colleagues (3.93), a problem that was affecting the very existence of these schools.[54] As Kenneth Ludmerer and other historians have pointed out, sectarian medicine had begun to decline in popularity as early as the 1890s. By the early twentieth century, with the advent of expensive innovations such as laboratory instruction and clinical clerkships, many of the sectarian schools, which were often proprietary and ran

Table 5.2 Wisconsin medical graduates, post-1905: The ten most frequently attended medical schools (*n* = 220, total *n* = 308)

School	Location	No. of graduates	% of total
Marquette	Milwaukee	79	25.6
Rush	Chicago	36	11.7
Wisconsin Physicians & Surgeons	Milwaukee	23	7.5
Northwestern	Chicago	21	6.8
Chicago Physicians & Surgeons	Chicago	19	6.2
Chicago Medical & Surgical	Chicago	12	3.9
University of Illinois	Chicago	10	3.2
Milwaukee Medical	Milwaukee	8	2.6
Bennett	Chicago	7	2.3
Hahnemann	Chicago	5	2.0

Sources: Louis Frederick Frank, "Directory of Milwaukee Physicians, 1834–1914," *The Medical History of Milwaukee, 1834–1914* (Milwaukee: Germania Publishing Co., 1915), pp. 238–271; also Board of Medical Examiners, Physician Licenses (Series 1606) and Register of Physicians (Series 1621), Archives Division, Wisconsin State Historical Society, Madison, Wisconsin.

on extremely lean budgets, closed their doors, unable to afford the equipment or staff necessary for modern medical education.[55]

The curricular improvements for the orthodox medical schools in the Midwest, however, had not come without a heavy price. Indeed, for the Milwaukee schools between 1906 and 1914, these new standards threatened their very existence. Forced by adverse reports of the American Medical Association's Council on Medical Education, both schools upgraded their entrance requirements, added more laboratory science, and increased the amount of time students spent in the hospital.[56] But despite the addition of laboratories and other improvements at the Milwaukee Medical College and at the Wisconsin College of Physicians and Surgeons, when Abraham Flexner visited the schools in February 1910, he excoriated both of them. He reported that the Milwaukee Medical College possessed only "meager facilities" for teaching pathology and bacteriology, and the equipment for the experimental physiology and toxicology courses was "slight." Milwaukee Medical College's clinical facilities were "extremely weak." Teaching at this school was "limited to amphitheater clinics." At the Wisconsin College of Physicians and Surgeons, though the "room given to histology and pathology [was] clean . . . adequate to routine elementary work," most of the laboratory facilities were reported to be like those of anatomy, which he described as "very poor; there is not even a complete skeleton." The clinical facilities at this school were even worse than those across town. Flexner reported that Wisconsin P&S had "utterly wretched" clinical facilities: "the school gives amphitheater clinics only." In his general consideration of medical education in Wisconsin, Flexner concluded that "the two Milwaukee schools are without a redeeming feature . . . Neither of the schools meets the most lenient standards."[57]

Within the next three years, further reviews by national medical accrediting groups pushed these schools over the edge of survival. In 1911 and 1912, the AMA's Council on Medical Education ranked both schools as Class B—that is, both needed major overhauls to come up to acceptable standards. In its third report, for the school year 1913, the AMA council was prepared to issue each school a Class C rating, which would have precluded licensure of the schools' graduates in most states. When news of this development leaked out to the students at Milwaukee Medical College, they revolted and left the school to enroll at the Wisconsin College of Physicians and Surgeons, where it was understood "that action would be taken immediately to make changes required to obtain a higher rating."[58]

With the Milwaukee Medical College effectively defunct, Marquette University was relieved of its nominal affiliation with a medical school. However, the medical community was aware that a medical school in the city would have to have university affiliation in order to survive. Within several months, they helped Marquette University to purchase outright the Wisconsin College of Physicians and Surgeons and to lease the buildings of the old Milwaukee Medical College. The effective union of the two schools under the direct control of Marquette University brought to Milwaukee what had become the American model of modern medical education: university control of medical education. With the university's backing, the Marquette Medical School hired four full-time professors in the preclinical sciences and began to build close affiliations for clinical work at several of the city's large hospitals. By 1915, the Council on Medical Education acknowledged the school's significant reforms and gave it a Class A rating.[59]

The Chicago schools attended by Wisconsin students after 1905 also increased their admission requirements. Rush Medical College, still popular among Wisconsin students because it was a major recipient of graduates from the two-year program at the University of Wisconsin Medical School, began to require two years of college preparation in 1904. Northwestern University followed a few years later, requiring a year of college in 1908 and two years in 1911. By making courses such as chemistry and physics, which had previously been taught in the first year, a prerequisite for admission instead, Rush and Northwestern were able to consolidate preclinical subjects into the first two years in an attempt to improve the clinical time offered junior and senior medical students.[60]

The training for the 308 Wisconsin physicians who registered between 1906 and 1928 reflected an increasing emphasis on hospital experience. Breaking this subsample into three time periods, Figures 5.1, 5.2, and 5.3 illustrate the gradual evolution in the amount of clinical time spent in the hospital. For the 116 doctors who registered between 1906 and 1909, though the mean number of months of hospital training equaled 6.01, over half of the doctors in training had not spent any clinical time in the hospital. The 164 physicians in the

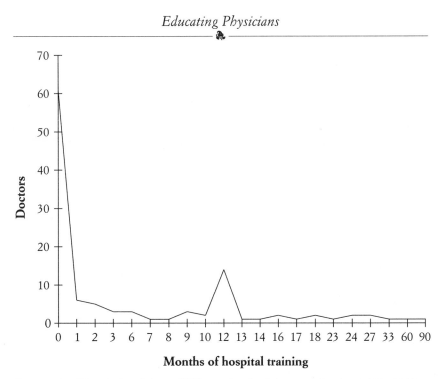

Figure 5.1   Hospital training of Wisconsin physicians graduating 1906–1909 (*n* = 116)

group of registrants between 1910 and 1919 had only slightly more hospital time (the mean was now 6.88), and 65 of them (40.6 percent of known cases) still had no hospital instruction. The number of doctors in the post-1920 group (28) may be small, but it shows a dramatic increase in the clinical time spent in the hospital: the mean number of months was 10.65; and only 6 doctors (23.1 percent of known cases) had never had any hospital time, while 19 (72.9 percent of known cases) had between one and twelve months of hospital experience. The trend was not universal, however. At Rush, for example, the post-1905 group spent almost five more months in the hospital than the pre-1905 group did: the earlier group had a mean of 5.63 months, the later group's mean was 10.05.[61] But at Northwestern University Medical School until well after World War I, senior medical students still spent some clinical time at amphitheater clinics.[62]

Despite these demonstrable improvements in the rigor and the content of medical education by the turn of the twentieth century, however, improvements in obstetric education lagged behind other cur-

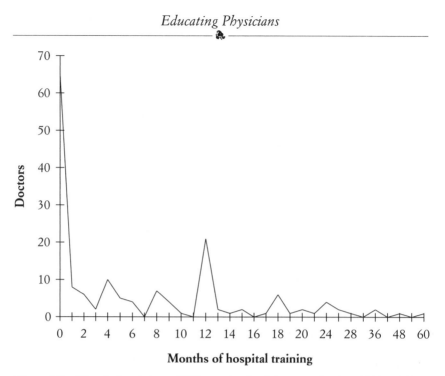

Figure 5.2 Hospital training of Wisconsin physicians graduating 1910–1919 (*n* = 164)

ricular reforms. Indeed, in his 1910 report on American medical schools, Abraham Flexner singled out obstetrics, among all of the clinical subjects, for particularly harsh criticism. He pronounced didactic lectures as "utterly worthless" and the manikin "of value only to a limited degree." The practice of obstetrics, he maintained, "is a fine art which cannot be picked up in the exigencies of out-patient work, poorly supervised at that. Principles, methods, technique, can be learned and skill acquired only in an adequately equipped maternity hospital."[63] He noted that many medical schools provided very little hospital obstetrical experience and that at seven schools, obstetrics was "practically altogether out-patient work." Students at these schools, Flexner asserted, got "about the same training as a midwife."[64]

Two years after Flexner's report, J. Whitridge Williams published the results of his survey of obstetrical departments in American medical schools.[65] Though the schools that responded were about evenly divided in merit, the quality of the obstetrical training offered by these

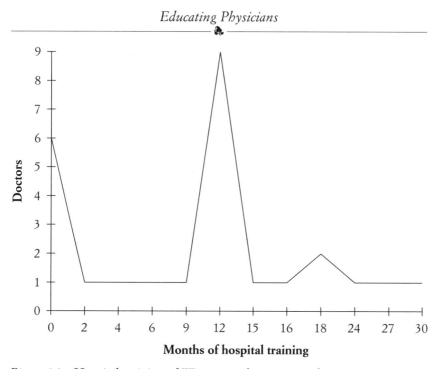

Figure 5.3 Hospital training of Wisconsin physicians graduating 1920–1930 (*n* = 28)

schools did not correspond to their overall standing.[66] Elite medical schools reported as many problems with their obstetrical training as the eleven "not acceptable" ones.[67]

Williams questioned each department about the training of its obstetrics professors (including their ability to do operative obstetrics), the clinical facilities available for teaching, the relationship of the department to the school's gynecologic service, the quality of both the school's students and their obstetrics training upon graduation, the extent of midwife practice in the community where the school was located, and the department's recommendations for improving obstetrical training and practice in general. In presenting his survey results, Williams acknowledged that "for many years I have regarded the general attitude toward obstetrical teaching as a very dark spot in our system of medical education, and the majority of the replies to my questionnaire indicate that my pessimism was more than justified."[68]

The results of Williams' survey presented a doleful picture of ob-

stetrical teaching in American medical schools. Over one-third of obstetrics professors in his survey were not strictly specialists—they did
not limit their practice solely to obstetrics and gynecology. Only about
half of Williams's sample had deliberately set out to become professors of obstetrics; the other half admitted that chance alone had conferred on them their post. As a result, many professors' preparation
was quite limited. Only nine professors out of forty-three had seen a
thousand or more cases of labor; five had seen fewer than a hundred
cases; one acknowledged that he had never seen a woman delivered
before he assumed his professorship. Several professors admitted that
they were not competent to perform major operations, including cesarean sections. One-fourth of the professors, including three from
elite medical schools, conceded that they could not care for some
major obstetrical complications, such as extrauterine pregnancies.

In addition to poorly trained obstetrics professors, most of the
schools in Williams's survey had very limited obstetrics facilities. Only
nine schools had hospitals with adequate clinical facilities for teaching
obstetrics, twenty-eight were inadequate in some major way, and six
had no connection at all with lying-in hospitals. Calculating the ratio
of students to deliveries, Williams found that in over half of the
schools in his survey (25 of 43), each student saw three or fewer cases
of childbirth—too few, in Williams's opinion, for satisfactory instruction in obstetrics. Only eight schools gave students the opportunity
to witness five or more cases, five being the minimum Williams
thought necessary. Though by this period many of the schools offered
outpatient delivery services, Williams discounted this type of clinical
training as a useful gauge of the adequacy of an obstetrics program
because the mere number of women cared for did not give a sufficient
measure of the school's teaching potential. As Williams pointed out,
"In order to be efficient for teaching, an outpatient service must be
held in rigid discipline, be organized as an integral part of the regular
obstetric service, and conducted through the lying-in hospital. Moreover, the students should not be sent to the homes of the patients
alone, but should always be accompanied by an assistant to demonstrate the case, as well as by a trained nurse."[69]

Asked to consider whether or not graduates from their schools were
competent to practice obstetrics upon graduation, about one-quarter
of the professors in Williams's survey answered no. Of the remaining

professors who thought overall that their students were proficient, many qualified their answers by saying that some of their students were competent or that their students could at least handle normal labor. Commenting on his own school, Williams acknowledged that even Johns Hopkins students were "unfit on graduation to practice obstetrics in its broad sense, and [were] scarcely prepared to handle normal cases."[70]

Summarizing his results, Williams found obstetrics education in even America's "acceptable" medical schools to be in a "deplorable condition." Many obstetrics professors, he observed, believed that general practitioners were equal in responsibility to midwives in causing deaths from puerperal fever. Indeed, many of these professors acknowledged that more childbearing women died from improper obstetrical operations than from infection caused by midwives. To remedy this appalling situation, Williams proposed seven reforms for obstetrics education. These included the recognition by medical schools of obstetrics as "one of the fundamental branches of medicine." The chair of the department needed to be a scientifically trained obstetrician who was a "real professor," and who concentrated solely on teaching and advancing knowledge; this person should not intend merely to be a "prosperous practitioner." General practitioners needed to be educated—to be made aware of their limitations and convinced that "major obstetrics is major surgery . . . [to] be undertaken only by specially trained men in control of abundant hospital facilities." To certify that physicians were adequately trained to attend childbirth, Williams demanded that state licensing boards require every applicant to submit proof that he or she had "seen delivered and has personally examined, under appropriate clinical conditions, at least ten women."[71]

J. Whitridge Williams has been credited with changing the teaching of obstetrics and gynecology in American medical schools in the first three decades of the twentieth century "from an empirical, technical craft to an academic discipline."[72] While some historians might argue that Joseph B. DeLee's work also had a profound influence on the teaching and practice of obstetrics,[73] most would agree on the long-term effects of Williams's influence on obstetrics. However, the problem is assessing Williams's influence in the years immediately following his report. The evidence regarding students who attended midwestern medical schools after 1910 shows only slow progress in the upgrading of obstetrics teaching from an "empirical, technical craft," at least when measured against Williams's criteria. But it is important to remember that Williams's ultimate goal in setting standards was to lead obstetrics towards its own professional specialization. Midwestern medical schools found themselves unable to meet these new standards.

After 1915, students at midwestern medical schools did begin to attend more births, both in the hospital and at women's homes.[74] Improvements in obstetrics teaching, even at the best medical schools, however, lagged behind many of the other clinical specialties. In 1934, the chair of the obstetrics department at the University of Michigan Medical School, Dr. Norman Miller, documented the problems with his program.[75] He pointed out that Michigan students received sufficient training in the theory and fundamentals of obstetrics, but he acknowledged that his students' clinical training did not even meet the Michigan State Board of Registration requirement of six deliveries per student.[76] Of Michigan's 1934 senior class, 25 percent had never attended a single delivery, 60 percent had attended one or two births, and only 15 percent had witnessed three or four births. To improve obstetrics training, Miller embarked on a fund-raising campaign to increase the number of charity patients in the university's maternity hospital, and managed by 1936 to raise the number of deliveries there by 62 percent. But Miller's problems with teaching obstetrics continued. Even by the 1940s, the obstetrics department faced the problem of having not enough patients.[77]

Wisconsin's medical leaders, like those in Michigan, also sought to improve the obstetrical training of their medical students. Within two years of the publication of Flexner's report and in the same year as Williams's survey, the Wisconsin State Board of Medical Examiners mandated that all new applicants for Wisconsin licenses present evidence of having attended at least six births "under proper supervision." Though the board does not appear to have strictly required each applicant to report on his or her obstetrical training (over 54 percent of the licensees had no information on their obstetrical training), the mean number of cases attended by graduation did rise, from 20.64 for the period 1910–1919 to 30.68 for the period 1920–1930. The median number of cases (that is, the number of cases attended by the person at the halfway point of the sample) also rose, from fifteen to twenty.[78] (See Figures 5.4 and 5.5.)

But the concern of Wisconsin's medical leaders about obstetrical training did not extend in the direction of academic obstetrics as defined by J. Whitridge Williams. Instead, both in the planning of the University of Wisconsin Medical School and in later attempts to establish postgraduate training through county medical societies, physicians in Wisconsin consciously sought to improve the training of general practitioners. This attempt was arguably more successful in the long run in convincing the public of the scientific expertise of all physicians.

Planners for the University of Wisconsin Medical School showed concern for the teaching of clinical subjects such as obstetrics, but instead of attempting to create obstetrical specialists, they worked within a tradition of training general practitioners. When the university began its preparations for adding a third and fourth year to its program in the late 1920s, it hired full-time clinicians to teach medicine and surgery but hired only part-time clinicians to teach obstet-

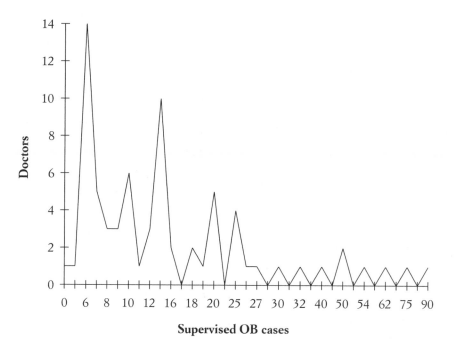

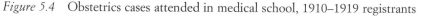

Figure 5.4 Obstetrics cases attended in medical school, 1910–1919 registrants

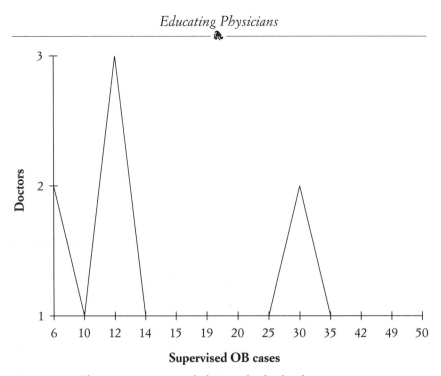

Figure 5.5 Obstetrics cases attended in medical school, 1920–1930 registrants

rics. The specialties, such as obstetrics, the Medical School decided, were to be taught from the general practitioner's point of view. Only one prominent Wisconsin physician debated the wisdom of this approach. Dorothy Reed Mendenhall wrote, "If the care of the obstetric patient by the average physician is inadequate it merely reflects the poor training he received while a medical student. Medical faculties have long talked about the lack of facilities and time for the proper instruction in obstetrics but very little has been done to improve the situation." She criticized the University of Wisconsin Medical School for hiring only part-time professors for obstetrics and gynecology and argued that "obstetrics and gynecology should form a major subject in the clinical curriculum" because family physicians might at any time have to "meet an obstetrical emergency of major importance under conditions which would appall the specialist who works only in a well equipped maternity."[79]

Dorothy Reed Mendenhall's criticism of medical school education in obstetrics was not echoed by other Wisconsin medical leaders.[80]

Mendenhall, unlike most of the state's leading physicians, had trained at Johns Hopkins and then gone on to do postdoctoral laboratory research. In the early twentieth century, she worked with the Children's Bureau, surveying childbearing conditions in the United States and Europe.[81] Despite, or perhaps because of, their lack of extensive training in obstetrics, most Wisconsin physicians did not engage in the sometimes extremely critical assessment of the obstetric skills of the general practitioner leveled by national medical leaders like J. Whitridge Williams. Instead, Wisconsin's medical leaders, many of whom were themselves general practitioners, worked in other ways to increase and modernize the skills of the state's doctors.

An analysis of the *Transactions of the State Medical Society of Wisconsin* and the *Wisconsin Medical Journal,* which became the official journal of the state society in 1901, showed little evidence that the national debate about the need for specialized obstetrical training and specialists in obstetrics had extended to Wisconsin. They acknowledged the contributions of science to improving childbirth, but while the state's physicians felt free to criticize the work done by midwives, they were cautious in their criticism of fellow practitioners. Indeed, instead of criticizing general practitioners and attempting to push them out of practice, many leaders wrote of their concern for their very survival. As one physician wrote, "This [reform in medical education] has all been done in the interest of the public of tomorrow . . . What of the 140,000 workers of today? These men will bear the brunt of the fight for many years to come. Is it not worth while to try at least to give them better equipment, to teach them what is being developed in the quiet zone at the rear? Is the experienced soldier at the front to be forgotten in the training of the recruit?"[82]

One of the problems was how to provide more training for these "experienced soldiers." Medical leaders in the state urged family physicians to avail themselves of the opportunity to attend one of the many graduate medical programs for additional education, but they acknowledged the difficulties most practicing doctors faced in attending these courses. As Rock Sleyster, a suburban Milwaukee practitioner and the editor of the *Wisconsin Medical Journal,* explained, "The greater number of practitioners are . . . unable, for financial, business or other reasons, to leave their homes and practice for a sufficient length of time to take up resident graduate work at any of these schools."[83] The solution, as Sleyster and others saw it, was to develop a graduate medical program through the University of Wisconsin Extension Division for demonstration lectures and correspondence study. Thus, instead of excluding some practitioners as unprofessional, they attempted to bring scientific competence to the entire profession.

When the legislature approved funding of the graduate medical extension courses in 1917, the State Medical Society began offering several courses for the state's physicians. Developed along lines of its popular "Farmers' Institutes," in which university scientists and other experts would take the train into rural counties and set up demonstrations and lectures for several days, the extension courses offered films and lectures by prominent physicians in addition to correspondence study. In 1922, after visits to some of the leading European obstetrical clinics, physicians working with the Extension began offering a postgraduate course in obstetrics using a number of films and lantern slides obtained from clinics in Vienna, London, and New York that illustrated the physiology of labor, difficult obstetrical procedures, and even the technique of cesarean section under local anesthesia. Four prominent Wisconsin obstetricians led the several day-long courses.[84] Designed to be given to members of county medical societies, the course was meant to acquaint country doctors with the latest obstetrical techniques. While several county societies did schedule this course for their members, editorials in the *Wisconsin Medical Journal* throughout the 1920s complained that not enough physicians were availing themselves of the opportunity to take advantage of these extension courses. The editors admonished the state's doctors, noting that the opportunity for postgraduate study had been "brought to our very door." Physicians were told that "the best way to increase one's income is to turn the key in the office door as often as possible and take postgraduate work. For the people soon know why you are away."[85]

But even as Wisconsin's medical leaders saw a place for general practitioners and tried to encourage them to obtain more training in obstetrics, national leaders in the field were moving to restrict practice and to establish obstetrics as a specialty. In 1930, the American Medical Association's Section on Obstetrics, together with the American Association of Obstetricians and Gynecologists and the American Gynecological Society, agreed to establish a specialty board in obstetrics and gynecology. Seeking a curb on obstetrical procedures performed by general practitioners, particularly obstetrical surgery, founders of the American Board of Obstetrics and Gynecology sought to establish educational and practice credentials for specialty practice. But strict educational requirements, at least for the first several years, were not rigorously enforced. Until 1932, prestigious and recognized obstetricians were admitted as founders; physicians with ten years of full-time experience in obstetrics and gynecology were admitted after passing an examination covering practical, oral, bedside, clinical, and laboratory aspects of the subject. Only recent specialists were required to have formal education in obstetrics: they had to have had three years of postgraduate training and to have practiced for at least two years as a specialist. The board also stringently enforced the meaning of specialization: no physician, regardless of training, could accept other than women patients. Thus, even well-trained general practitioners were excluded from board certification. In addition, the board sought to restrict general practitioner activities in the field by limiting hospital appointments in obstetrics to board members only. By the mid-1930s, the medical and lay public, including hospital directors, it was claimed, used board certification as a means of determining competence in a specialty.[86]

Had these strict rules governing obstetrical practice become part of state licensure requirements, they could have placed a considerable restraint on Wisconsin physicians' practice. As this chapter has shown, Wisconsin physicians even by 1930 had only meager training in obstetrics, and few practitioners had any advanced work in the field. Furthermore, there were few opportunities within the state to do advanced work in obstetrics. The University of Wisconsin Medical School had only a small residency program, the only one in the state throughout the 1930s.[87] Indeed, there were only 167 residency programs in either obstetrics or gynecology throughout the United States in 1930, though this number had increased to 269 by 1940.[88] In addition to difficulties in obtaining advanced training, most Wisconsin physicians could not afford to limit their practice solely to obstetrics:

there simply were not enough deliveries in the small towns and rural areas where many of the state's physicians practiced to maintain a board-defined "specialty" practice. For most of the state's physicians, therefore, obstetrics remained one of the many facets of a traditional general practice.[89] The next chapter analyzes the pace and the locale of the obstetrical practice of some of these general practitioners.

CHAPTER SIX

Country Doctors Replace Midwives

"No young or old physician settles in a new locality in the country who does not almost the first call meet with a case of obstetrics," wrote Dr. W. T. Sarles of Sparta, Wisconsin, in 1894.[1] Indeed, he argued, "if a country doctor should be a specialist in one branch of the science of medicine more than another it should be in that of obstetrics. Nothing will try his skill and patience more thoroughly and more often than this one department of his chosen profession. Many of the most prominent and vivid experiences in the professional lives of you who have seen ten, twenty or forty years of general practice in the country, has been in this department of medicine."[2]

In the late nineteenth and early twentieth centuries, many Wisconsin doctors shared Dr. Sarles's experiences as a country doctor. Indeed, it could be argued that rural general practice was the dominant model in the state until well into the twentieth century. Though increasing numbers of medical school graduates in this period were deciding to try their luck with an urban medical practice, many Wisconsin medical graduates, more than half of whom had been born in the state, returned to practice medicine in the small country towns where they had grown up.[3] Furthermore, as noted in the last chapter, though some medical schools were moving to train specialists who would establish urban practices, the University of Wisconsin Medical School made a conscious decision to keep training general practitioners.[4]

Over the course of the fifty years between 1870 and 1920, doctors attended childbirth in increasing numbers, and rural general practitioners were the first to assume the increasing numbers of maternity cases formerly handled by midwives. This chapter examines the transition from midwife to physician-assisted childbirth by analyzing the changes over time in the obstetrical practice of these country doctors. Milwaukee physicians, by contrast, seemed to eschew obstetrical cases. Only about a quarter of Milwaukee physicians in practice in 1885 had obstetrical cases, a figure that rose only slightly, to 32 percent, by 1895.[5] Indeed, overall, Milwaukee physicians in the sample delivered an average of only 1.36 babies per month, while the doctors from the rural counties attended a monthly average of 2.77 births.[6] The situation in Milwaukee was typical: as late as 1907, a survey of Cleveland physicians found that midwives continued to oversee most deliveries; doctors were called only when midwives encountered unusual difficulty.[7] However, as the next chapter will show, by the second decade of the twentieth century, urban physicians were the ones who became obstetrical specialists.

This change in birth attendants at the end of the nineteenth century occurred at the same time that many American medical schools were attempting to reform their curricula. Though many Midwestern medical schools were slow to introduce the curricular reforms that were part of the new emphasis on scientific medicine, physicians who began their practice in Wisconsin after the turn of the twentieth century were better educated than before. Indeed, in Wisconsin, as elsewhere, physicians claimed that this improved, scientific training gave them new authority to make decisions about such health matters as those relating to maternity.[8]

The congruence of dates between the improvement of doctors' medical education and their assumption of obstetrical cases naturally raises the question of whether the public, specifically birthing women, turned to physician birth attendants because of this better training. As Judith Walzer Leavitt has demonstrated, early in the nineteenth century some women sought out physicians because they believed that these doctors offered some relief from the fear of death and debility related to childbirth.[9] Yet, as this chapter demonstrates, this trend to physician-assisted childbirth was not an embracing of a distinct medical specialist who represented the model of a disembodied, objective, ideal science. Instead, as the analysis of the geographic and demographic factors of the practice of these doctors shows, physicians' obstetrical practice, like those of the midwives, were built by ties based on class, ethnicity, and geography.[10] Thus, though the Progressive period has been characterized by its espousing of what Paul Starr calls the "legitimate complexity of science," the analysis of physicians' obstetrical practice suggests that this science was adopted within a social context.[11]

Obstetrics Becomes Part of General Practice

Though Dr. Sarles wanted to claim obstetrics as the country doctor's specialty, the evidence from Wisconsin shows that for doctors who practiced in the 1870s and 1880s, obstetric cases formed only a small part of their practice (see Figure 6.1). Indeed, as described in Chapter 1, some doctors turned over their maternity cases to midwives, appearing in the birthing room only when the case was beyond the midwife's skills.[12] For the busy and entrepreneurial physician, obstetrical cases often claimed significant portions of time, time that could

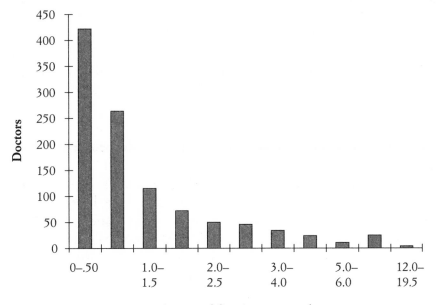

Average deliveries per month

Figure 6.1   Average number of physician-assisted deliveries per month, 1870–1920

be spent treating more patients whose fees exceeded those garnered in maternity cases.[13]

The limited obstetrical practice of George N. Hidershide, a physician in Trempealeau County, was typical. Dr. Hidershide, described in a county history as "dean of the medical profession in Trempealeau County, pioneer physician, retired army officer, useful citizen, and man-of-affairs,"[14] established a practice in Arcadia in 1875, shortly after the railroad was laid through the county. While he was celebrated for his "long and dreary rides by day and night, in summers' heat and winter's cold, through flood and drought, through snow and mud, through rain and hail," he undertook few of these rides to attend obstetrical cases. Though he practiced throughout the period under study, he attended only three deliveries in 1877, none in 1880 and 1885, only one in 1890, three in 1895, and none in 1900. By 1905, he began to attend a few more births per year, but with the exception of 1915, he never attended more than two or three births in a six-month period.[15]

Like Dr. Hidershide, many nineteenth century rural physicians did not take on obstetrical cases when they began their medical practice (see Figure 6.2).[16] Despite the accepted wisdom that only young practitioners took on childbirth cases, of the eight doctors in Trempealeau and Price counties who began their practice between 1886 and 1890, four waited five or more years before they began to attend births. Six doctors out of twelve who began in the years between 1891 and 1895 did not deliver a baby until at least 1905.[17]

Yet, as early as the decade of the 1890s, physicians in two rural counties of this study oversaw more than half of the deliveries in their area, and by 1900, young physicians were much more likely than before to begin their practice including obstetrical cases. Between 1906 and 1910, in fact, only one of the seven physicians who began practice in these rural counties delayed accepting maternity patients.[18] Indeed, by then obstetrics was becoming an integral part of a general practice for both young and more established physicians. By 1920, almost all the physicians listed in various medical directories were found to be delivering babies. Table 6.1 illustrates the rise in number of physician-assisted deliveries for Trempealeau and Price Counties.[19]

That Wisconsin's physicians, especially general practitioners, took on obstetrical cases at the beginning of the twentieth century contrasts

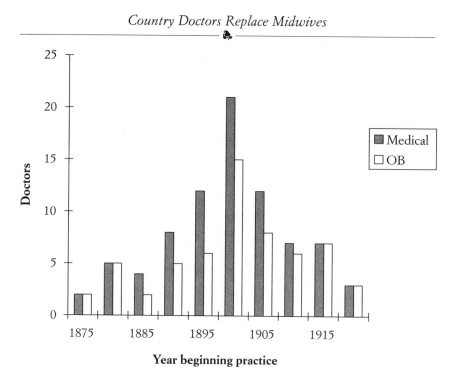

Figure 6.2 Rural physicians beginning obstetrical practice within five years of beginning practice

Table 6.1 Trempealeau and Price County physicians: Numbers of physicians attending childbirths and average number of deliveries per year

Year	No. of physicians attending childbirth	Mean no. of deliveries per year
1877	10	5.20
1880	8	19.75
1885	15	14.27
1890	15	16.00
1895	18	15.44
1900	39	15.97
1905	40	13.93
1910	42	14.83
1915	43	17.51
1920	40	23.55

Sources: Sampled birth records, 1877–1920: Birth Records, Trempealeau and Price Counties, Wisconsin Vital Records Office, Wisconsin Department of Health and Human Services, Madison, Wisconsin.

with the findings of at least one historian, who stated, "By the late 1920s, even in rural areas, the general practitioner no longer attempted major surgery and had often given up the practice of obstetrics, nose and throat diseases, and venereal diseases."[20] Rather, as the figures in Table 6.1 show, despite the worries of turn-of-the-century medical leaders about the problems of attracting physicians to rural maternity care, an increased proportion of doctors in Trempealeau and Price County added obstetrics to their general practice.[21] By 1920, in fact, physicians in these areas of rural Wisconsin actually had increased the number of deliveries per month that they attended.

Dr. Charles D. Fenelon, the physician with the largest sampled obstetrical practice in Price County, exemplified the country practitioners who built active obstetrical practices in rural Wisconsin around 1900. Born in Wisconsin, Dr. Fenelon received a college degree and then took a two-year preceptorship prior to attending Rush Medical School, where he received his medical degree in 1891. Perhaps seeing an opportunity to build a medical practice where there was little competition, he moved to the small Price County town of Phillips soon after graduation from medical school.[22] Like many physicians, Fenelon was also involved in the drugstore business. By 1895, he was co-owner of a drug store with E. D. Sperry, the brother of the only other doctor in Phillips. Dr. Fenelon quickly built his practice, accepting many maternity cases so that in 1900, he attended sixty-three births, the most of any doctor in Price County. Twenty years later, in 1920, Dr. Fenelon was still practicing medicine in the county, but perhaps due either to his age or to competition from other colleagues, he attended only forty-two births that year.[23]

Paul Starr has suggested that the "transportation revolution" of the nineteenth century, together with the advent of the telephone, helped to create a much larger market for physician services by helping to lower what he terms the "indirect prices" of medical care.[24] This reduction of indirect costs in turn allowed physicians to become more productive and to make a full-time living practicing medicine. The late nineteenth-century physician thus could expect to support a family by a medical practice.[25] But how much of a role did this "transportation revolution" play in the increase in the number of physicians attending obstetrical cases in rural Wisconsin?

As the quote describing Dr. Hidershide made clear, transportation difficulties played a large role in a nineteenth-century rural physician's practice. Maternity cases could be a particular problem, because a woman might contact the doctor only when she was in active labor, or when something had gone wrong, and physicians would be left with very little time to get to their patients. Dr. L. G. Armstrong, the rural physician who commented on Dr. Sarles's paper, characterized the typical situation:

> In the great majority of cases they [rural patients] fail to let you know anything about your being required until the woman gives the alarm that labor has commenced. Then if a speedy horse can get the messenger to you, and you back to the patient in time, you have a chance to do something; . . . If you arrive there in good time to render that assistance which is always absolutely necessary, why you have done well. But on the other hand, if you are there . . . after the work is mainly over . . . you find all of the terrible conditions which [a previous speaker] has portrayed.[26]

Even by 1920, as C. M. Schuldt, a Platteville, Wisconsin, physician, asserted, "the difficulty in traveling consumes much of the energy which he [the doctor] needs in caring for his patients." Bad roads were dangerous, he noted, so that "people cannot expect the physician to come day or night, regardless of weather, since he, too, is only human and needs to look out for his own welfare as well as others."[27]

Poor roads and the isolation of rural life also limited the kind of help a country doctor doing obstetrics could summon in an emergency. Doctors delivering babies in the country had to be self-sufficient and well prepared. Describing a hypothetical case of postpartum hemorrhage, a Sharon, Wisconsin, physician communicated the tension undoubtedly shared by most of his colleagues. Cases like this were particularly difficult, he wrote, for "you [the doctor] may be ten miles from another physician and with only untried help to assist you."[28] B. J. Wadey, a Belleville, Wisconsin, physician, ascribed the higher maternal mortality found in rural Wisconsin in the early decades of the twentieth century to the problems of transportation. He noted, "In rural communities the obstetrical outfit must be complete, as we must be prepared to meet with any type of case."[29] Comparing urban and rural obstetrics, he asserted that city physicians could leave a laboring woman in the care of a nurse, who would "call you only when needed." In the country, however, "when possibly we are miles from our patient, when we arrive we are expected to stay." An overly rushed physician might then be too eager to deliver the case and then get away. This potential for interference, Wadey believed, led to higher maternal mortality in country practice.[30]

But despite the improvement in transportation methods in the early twentieth century, and though more physicians were taking on obstetrical cases, the total number of cases each physician attended and the geographic extent of this practice remained limited. Dr. Fenelon's obstetrical practice was typical. Though he attended the largest number of obstetrical cases of any doctor in Price County between 1895 and 1920, most of his patients came from Phillips, where he also lived.[31] But Dr. Fenelon did not monopolize obstetrical practice in his village. Most of the maternity patients of Dr. Willis P. Sperry, who also lived in Phillips, also were local women.[32] While other Price County doctors did not have such localized practices, the placement of railroad lines in relation to their home seemed to define the limits of their practice. Dr. D. Parry lived in Prentice, which was at the center of both the Wisconsin Railroad and the Minneapolis and St. Paul Railroad, which ran east and west through the county. Though he delivered most of his cases in the village of Prentice, Dr. Parry's outlying cases were in the settlements east and west of Prentice that lay along the Minneapolis and St. Paul Railroad. Even by 1920, when roads in the county had presumably been created or improved, Dr. J. S. Francis of Keenan (a town along the Minneapolis and St. Paul) attended cases only in the towns along the same railroad line.[33] The few cases that Drs. Fenelon and Sperry attended outside of Phillips followed this pattern as well. Their cases were all located in settlements along the Wisconsin Railroad, which ran north and south of Phillips through the county. Neither doctor attended births in any of the towns that were east and west of Phillips, on indirect roads.[34]

While the frontier conditions of Price County even as late as 1920 might explain the limited obstetrical practice of doctors in this area, the imperceptible changes in the obstetrical practice of the Rowley family doctors in Dane County demonstrates the limitations of using the transportation revolution to explain the increase in physician-attended births. Beginning in the 1860s, Dr. Newman C. Rowley, and later his son Antinous A. Rowley, rode their horses, and later took their horse and carriage, in a defined circuit through the northwest quarter of the county.[35] When A. A. Rowley's son, Dr. A. G. Rowley, purchased an automobile in 1905, the geographic dimensions of his obstetrical practice did not change.[36] Though some medical journals described doctors with cars who reportedly were able to triple the number of house calls they made,[37] Dr. A. G. Rowley did not attend more births, nor did he go any further to care for a case, than he or his father had prior to 1905.[38] Even by 1910, none of the sixteen births Rowley attended were further away than the fourteen-mile radius he had covered prior to purchasing his automobile.[39]

Other rural Dane County physicians had equally limited obstetrical practices in the late nineteenth and even into the twentieth century. The 9 doctors in rural Dane County in 1880 delivered an average of 7.77 babies per year, all in areas adjacent to their own home villages. The number of physicians attending births increased in the following years, but the mean number of births these doctors attended per month or per year did not change. Though some physicians in these years attended more than the average, many doctors oversaw only a few births. In 1900, for example, there were 45 physicians attending childbirth, but the mean number of births was only 6.15 per year, and in 1910, 47 rural Dane County doctors attended an average of 10.8 births a year.[40] Just as the number of births per physician remained constant over time, the distances these physicians traveled in Dane County also remained constant. Like Dr. Rowley, other physicians in the county added obstetrical cases based in villages and farms near their own.[41]

Whether by horse and carriage, railroad, or automobile, late nineteenth- and early twentieth-century Wisconsin physicians certainly faced formidable obstacles from the weather and the terrain in getting to their parturient patients.[42] But even with the invention of the automobile and the telephone, early twentieth-century Wisconsin physicians practicing in rural areas did not significantly increase the number of patients they oversaw nor the geographic extent of their obstetrical practice. For rural physicians like Dr. Fenelon and the Rowley's, obstetrics was not the major focus of their general practice. Even the busiest physician in Price County, Dr. Fenelon, handled an average of just five births a month; and Dr. Rowley, the busiest rural doctor in Dane County, delivered an average of only three babies a month. How then can we account for the increased number of physicians attending women in childbirth? The answer lies with an understanding of how the ideals of science and professionalism, as epitomized by the general practitioner, were molded by the context of culture and community.

Ethnicity and the Physician as Birth Attendant

As detailed in the last chapter, between 1870 and 1930 Wisconsin's physicians graduated from medical school with increasing amounts of education. Though specific improvements in obstetrics education lagged behind those in other subjects, even late nineteenth-century medical school graduates could claim to understand and even to represent the new ideas of scientific medicine. But a skeptical public had to be convinced of the usefulness of these new ideas, and physicians returning to the communities where they had been born and/or raised made ideal emissaries.

Historians have argued that much nineteenth-century medical practice was built on close personal relationships between physicians and their patients. Experience and judgment were important qualities for the physician who wished to build a successful practice. But as both Charles E. Rosenberg and John Harley Warner have emphasized, therapeutic efficacy throughout much of the nineteenth century depended on a physician's long-term knowledge of his patients' personal history and experience.[43] As Rosenberg explains, "A physician who knew a family's constitutional idiosyncracies was necessarily a better practitioner for that family than one who enjoyed no such insight."[44] Thus, the successful doctor had to be an integral part of the community.

In rural Wisconsin in the late nineteenth and early twentieth centuries, general practitioners were indeed important members of their communities. Of 115 physicians in the three rural areas of this study who could be found in the census, 59 (51.3 percent) were born in Wisconsin.[45] Furthermore, though a number of historians have argued that nineteenth-century physicians enjoyed very little respect for their occupation, the evidence from rural Wisconsin shows that doctors in these areas actually wielded a significant amount of political and economic authority.[46] In Trempealeau County, for example, Dr. F. L. Lewis was a founding supervisor of the village of Arcadia, on land that was owned in part by Dr. Isaac A. Briggs.[47] George N. Hidershide, who began his practice in Trempealeau County in 1875, played an integral part in establishing a local bank. He also served as president of his village and president of the library board, helped to found the local telephone company, and also served as a Republican party delegate at the county and state levels.[48] Dr. E. A. Olson, who began his practice in 1877, helped to organize and was the first president of the Osseo town council. He went on to serve as a Republican party delegate in district, county, and congressional conventions. Like Dr. Hidershide, Dr. Olson also helped found the local bank. He was also an active member of the Masons and the Knights of Pythias.[49] Henry A. Jegi began his practice in the county in 1897, and in addition to many public health duties, he became deeply involved in the Trempealeau County Board of Education. Like the other doctors, he was also a prominent bank stockholder and member of a number of fraternal organizations.[50] Dr. A. K. Olsen was cited in a county history as a "well-known and popular citizen, and with his family moves in the best society in this part of the country."[51]

The rise of the public health movement in the late nineteenth century extended the political and social influence of these physicians to the health concerns of their communities.[52] In rural Wisconsin, physicians who were already in positions of political authority helped to organize local departments of health. While health officers' reports show that they had only limited cooperation in enforcing the new ideas about public health, the job was important because it gave doctors the political authority within their own communities to espouse the ideas of professional science and medicine. Even if this job was largely symbolic, it carried a cultural authority linked, in many cases, to real political power, power that midwives did not share.[53]

Though most of the physicians practicing in the rural areas of this study were native born, nineteen doctors were European immigrants, the majority from Norway. Though most of these immigrant doctors received medical school diplomas from schools in the United States, their American education did not separate them from their immigrant communities. In fact, Dr. Hidershide, born in Luxembourg, did not learn to speak English until he apprenticed with a local doctor.[54] Dr.

A. K. Olsen came to the United States with a college degree from Norway. Three months after he received an M.D. from Rush Medical School in 1897, he moved to Ettrick, in Trempealeau County. Within months of this move, he married a Norwegian immigrant woman, and when she died, he married her sister.[55] Charles Van Hiddeson, a Dane County practitioner, lived in the German immigrant community in Sauk City, and Ole Mork, who came to the United States in 1908 with a Norwegian medical degree, settled in Trempealeau County with "many of his patients being his own countrymen".[56] Furthermore, though one Trempealeau County health officer complained in the 1880s of the difficulties in convincing immigrants to leave their "old world habits of life" in Europe,[57] both native-born and immigrant physicians in Trempealeau County served as health officers.[58]

The therapeutic necessity of close community doctor-patient relationships extended to maternity cases. While it undoubtedly is true that parturient women regarded physicians as having more knowledge and expertise than midwives, the ethnic bonds between Wisconsin physicians and their patients reveal that birthing women made their choices of expert help within certain parameters.[59] In rural Dane County in 1880, for example, six physicians, all born in North America, attended a total of 63 births. While over 30 percent of the county was foreign-born, over 81 percent of the patients of these doctors were American-born.[60]

At the same time, the immigrant doctors attended many more immigrant women than did their native-born colleagues, and the ethnic background of these physicians, together with their social and political positions within the Norwegian and native-born communities, helps to explain how late nineteenth-century general practitioners were able to displace midwives from the birthing room.[61] In Trempealeau County in 1900, for example, 50 percent of the obstetric patients of the three Norwegian doctors were Norwegian; for the fifteen American-born doctors, the percentage of Norwegian mothers averaged only 30 percent. The practice of Dr. E. A. Olson, of Trempealeau County, was typical of this group. Born in Norway, Dr. Olson came to Wisconsin as an infant in the 1850s. After graduating from a medical school in nearby Iowa in 1877, he returned to establish a practice in Arcardia in Trempealeau County, where he practiced at least through 1920.[62] Like many of the country doctors noted earlier in this chapter, his obstetrical practice did not begin to grow until the end of the nineteenth century, but many of his patients came from the sizable Norwegian community. Indeed, in 1895, eleven of his thirteen cases were Norwegian. Likewise, over 53 percent of the cases handled by Norwegian-born Dr. A. K. Olsen in 1900 were from Norwegian families, as were at least 65 percent of the maternity cases overseen by the more recent Norwegian immigrant physician Dr. Theodore Budom.[63]

The demographic dimensions of the obstetrical practice of Dr. Olsen and the others were typical of all of the immigrant doctors. Over all the years of the study, these Scandinavian physicians had significantly more Scandinavian patients than their American-born counterparts.[64] But the growing authority of physicians over childbirth in the immigrant community extended beyond this first generation of immigrant physicians. Among the rural physicians in this study, over half (58, or 50.5 percent) had parents who were not born in North America. For those twenty-three doctors who were ethnically Scandinavian, the bonds of community seemed especially strong.[65] In all the rural counties of this study, these physicians had significantly higher percentages of Scandinavian patients.[66]

At an 1894 meeting of the State Medical Society of Wisconsin, Dr. L. G. Armstrong decried the use of midwives among country families, but he also remarked that, in rural maternity cases, "it is now becoming more popular to have a physician."[67] This trend toward physician-assisted births accelerated by the beginning of the twentieth century. In fact, by 1915 only about 13 percent of all the births in Wisconsin were attended by midwives,[68] and most general practitioners found themselves overseeing at least a few deliveries a year. It seemed that the public was listening to physicians who argued that they were the scientific experts in matters of parturition.

Yet citing overall statistics that show a change from midwife- to physician-assisted childbirth blurs the important differences in this transition even within Wisconsin. Most births by 1910 in Trempealeau County were being overseen by physicians; but in Price County, midwives still prevailed. Why were there such differences, even though each county still had a high number of foreign-born families? The key, as the last part of this chapter has argued, lies in examining the social and cultural relationships between physicians and the communities where they practiced. Though at least nineteen of the rural doctors in this study were European immigrants, eleven of them lived in Trempealeau County and seven of them lived in Dane County. In Price County, on the other hand, though even as late as 1920 a sizable percentage of the population was foreign-born, only one immigrant doctor, O. A. Christenson, practiced there. Furthermore, of the nine Price County physicians with immigrant parents, only three came from non-English speaking backgrounds.[69] Thus, it is not surprising that the Swedish, Finnish, and German childbearing women of Price County, lacking a physician who could speak their language or understand their culture, continued to hire midwives to deliver their babies well into the twentieth century.[70]

In the small villages and towns of rural America in the late nineteenth and early twentieth centuries, physicians embodied both the old ideal of ethics and etiquette, as well as some of the new ideals of scientific medicine.[71] Midwives, on the other hand, no matter how they were trained, still practiced within a context shaped by gender and tradition. Yet despite the fact that by the end of the nineteenth century educational qualifications were increasingly important for professional success, ties to the community remained an important determinant of a successful medical practice.[72] In fact, the geographic and demographic contours of rural medical practice were strikingly similar to those of the midwives these doctors replaced. Physicians acted as emissaries of science, but the reception of these emissaries was conditioned by the social and political positions these doctors already occupied within the community.

By the early twentieth century, however, a new paradigm for medical practice was emerging in urban America. Specializing in one branch of medicine, some doctors were claiming a new professional model for medicine based in the laboratory and the hospital. As the next chapter will show, there were several paths toward specialism in obstetrics, including one that would accommodate the community-based practitioner. But as much as these general practitioners had pressed for physician-based maternity care, in the end, even they would find themselves eliminated from the birthing room.

CHAPTER SEVEN

Specializing Obstetrics

In a 1919 paper delivered to the American Medical Association's Section on Obstetrics, Gynecology and Abdominal Surgery, Dr. Henry P. Newman delineated some of the problems in defining obstetrics as a medical specialty. Obstetrics, he observed, was not like the other specialties that had "grown out of the advancement of the science of medicine, as research and study brought knowledge of disease manifestations." On the contrary, he pointed out, "with obstetrics one is not concerned with finding a new disease . . . but the safeguarding and superintending of what should be the most normal of all life functions." This difficulty with defining an area of expertise had further ramifications. According to Newman,

> Everybody is doing, has always done, obstetrics, and this continuity of common participation is one of the hardest things to break. In a short lifetime, with other, better defined, more recently organized specialties opening before him, the doctor hesitates to stake his future on a career in which associations are so indiscriminate and about which clings so much old custom and superstition of ignorance. One dislikes to be disputing the ground with midwives or poaching upon the broad preserves of the general practitioner.[1]

For urban, academic physicians like Drs. Newman, Joseph B. DeLee, and others, there were intellectual and even economic challenges to establishing obstetrics as a "scientific" medical specialty.

Midwives had been the easiest target. But the "midwife problem" was actually in decline; by 1915 midwife-attended births accounted for only 26 percent of all births in Milwaukee County.[2] Indeed, as noted in the last chapter, by the turn of the twentieth century, many physicians were adding obstetrical cases to their practices. But if a general practitioner could do obstetrics, the field could not claim a special base of knowledge. As one critic put it, "the middle class medical man, or general practitioner, so-called, is the greatest danger in obstetrics. A midwife, under strict control, does comparatively little harm, but the doctor who does obstetric work to get the medical practice of the family, . . . is the one responsible for many obstetric disasters."[3]

Though the majority of urban doctors in this period continued to practice general medicine, many of the accusations of the incompetence of general practitioners were directed at rural-based "country doctors." As Dr. Charles M. Ellis, the President of the Maryland Medical Society, asserted, "The greatest objection to the country doctor is that, as a rule, he takes a short course in medicine, and then is launched upon his field of labor without any further experience . . . The city and country doctor are supposed to be alike at the start, but the city doctor soon leaves the country one far behind." Indeed, he noted, a country practitioner could never aspire to greatness. "Men who are so successful rarely stay in the country. Like Sims, Agnew, Goodell, and others, they soon find their way to the large cities where they make their mark."[4] Though Wisconsin's physicians were as a rule more muted in their criticism of specifically country doctors, Dr. J. P. McMahon, Professor of Obstetrics at Marquette Medical School in Milwaukee, denounced general practitioners in his comments on a 1914 paper of puerperal fever as "inefficient professional male[s]" who did not understand that "obstetric practice is surgical practice, requiring surgical technique and experience."[5]

The attacks on rural general practitioners and the claims of physicians like McMahon and others for scientific medicine based in hospitals and medical schools eventually had enormous consequences for the practice of obstetrics. By the second half of the twentieth century, most births in the United States would take place in hospitals, overseen by obstetricians, who would claim a specific and specialized basis for their practice. Almost all of these specialists would be located in urban areas, leaving rural women no choice but to travel many miles to obtain care. Indeed, there were fewer doctors practicing in Trempealeau and Price Counties in the last part of the twentieth century than there had been in 1900.[6]

But in the early decades of the twentieth century this specialized view of obstetrics had not achieved the dominant position it would later occupy. Indeed, obstetricians, like midwives, were facing a crisis of professionalization. In Wisconsin, and in Milwaukee in particular, while some doctors advocated a new model of scientific obstetrics, other physicians claimed expertise in obstetrics based on the more traditional criterion of experience with patients. But like the busy urban midwives whose skills had been developed by overseeing many deliveries, these traditionally defined specialists lacked the institutional bases of support that came to define the professional healer in the twentieth century. By the 1930s, like the midwives and general practitioners before them, these experience-based specialists were superseded by doctors who claimed a specialism based in the hospital.

Taking on Maternity Cases: General Practitioners in Milwaukee

Though obstetric specialism in the twentieth century came to be associated with urban physicians, until the first decades of the twentieth century, many physicians in Milwaukee eschewed maternity cases. Indeed, as Dr. E. F. Fish contended in 1903, "for many years this branch of medicine has seemingly been relegated to the midwives and young practitioners in medicine; the older men fight shy of it, they do not seem to want it."[7]

Figure 7.1 demonstrates that Dr. Fish had not exaggerated about the extent of physician-directed maternity practice in nineteenth-century Milwaukee. Between 1873 and 1895, less than a third of all Milwaukee physicians in practice delivered babies.[8] This situation began to change around the turn of the twentieth century. Between 1895 and 1900, many more Milwaukee physicians began to include obstetrics in their general practice. By 1910, almost 60 percent of the city's doctors had performed a delivery, double the percentage of only twenty years before. However, for most urban practitioners, the movement into obstetrical practice in the first few years of the twentieth century was not a movement towards specialization in the field.

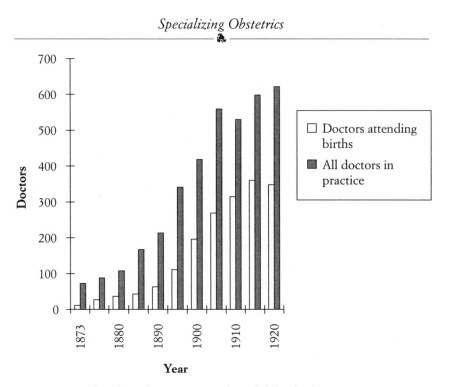

Figure 7.1   Milwaukee physicians attending childbirths, by year

As Figure 7.2 shows, even by 1920, the average Milwaukee physician who took maternity cases attended between two and three births per month. Furthermore, like the cases of both rural doctors and urban midwives, the obstetrical cases of most Milwaukee doctors generally came from their own neighborhood, though there were some changes over time. These phenomena are best seen by analyzing the obstetrical practices of Milwaukee doctors in 1880, 1900, and 1920.

Within a four-month period in 1880, 34 physicians attended one or more births in Milwaukee. As Figure 7.2 shows, the mean number of deliveries per month was small. Indeed, the doctor with the largest obstetrical practice in Milwaukee County in this period, Dr. Anton Hirshbuehl, who attended sixteen births in a four-month period, lived outside of Milwaukee in the small, rural village of Bayview.[9] Like the midwives of this period, all the doctors who attended births delivered women who lived either in their own wards or in wards contiguous to their own. Professional affiliations made little difference. Even Robert Martin, who became the city's Commissioner of Health in 1881, attended only seven births over a three-month period, all in

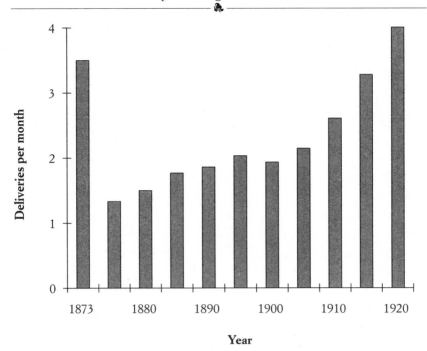

Figure 7.2 Milwaukee physicians: Mean number of deliveries per month, by year

areas near his home. Three of his women patients lived in his own fifth ward, the remaining cases were based in adjacent wards.[10]

Even busy doctors—those physicians who attended a total of at least ten births in all of the sampled years—did not go far from home to assist at a delivery.[11] Despite the probability that many of these physicians were undoubtedly called out to assist at difficult deliveries that midwives could not handle, the locality index for the eleven busy doctors in 1880 was 0.424, a number lower than the 1873 busy midwife index of 0.55.[12]

By 1900, though many more doctors in Milwaukee were overseeing obstetrical cases, neither the average number of cases per month each practitioner assumed nor the geographic parameters of their practice increased dramatically. As Figure 7.2 shows, the mean number of deliveries per doctor in 1900 had increased slightly from the 1880 level, from about 1.5 to 2.0. But few physicians deviated very far from this mean: only nine doctors attended five or more births per month, and no doctor attended more than an average of eight deliveries per month.[13] Indeed, even Dr. Fish, who was listed as a Fellow of the American Association of Obstetrics and Gynecology, attended only three births in a three-month period.[14] Though the 1900 locality index for the busiest physicians (1.320) exceeded that of the midwives in practice in that year (0.99), it showed that most physicians still were going to births only one or two wards beyond the confines of their own home ward.[15] Thus, for the 141 physicians whose home ward could be determined, almost 55 percent ($n = 77$) still attended births either in their own ward or in one that was contiguous. Furthermore, 34 other doctors could also be considered neighborhood practitioners, as their patients lived in the same districts, though not in contiguous wards. Only 30 doctors in the 1900 sample (21.3 percent) left their neighborhoods to attend a birth.

Though it would be tempting to portray these 30 doctors as a sort of vanguard of obstetrical professionalism, the explanations for their willingness to travel across the city were probably idiosyncratic and did not anticipate a specialist practice. Thus, doctors with larger practices were as likely as those with small obstetrical caseloads to attend a birth close to home.[16] For example, Dr. C. H. Lewis, living in the seventeenth ward on the city's South Side, had one of the smallest indices (0.462) and one of the largest practices (twenty-four deliveries in three months); and H. S. Piggins, who attended twenty-two births in three months, traveled no further in the south side than Joseph Dries, who attended only one birth in the same period.[17] Though electric trolley lines were providing reasonable public transportation across the city by 1900, no one group of medical practitioners took advantage of this improvement in transportation.[18]

By 1920, Milwaukee physicians were attending significantly more births per month on average than they had at the turn of the twentieth century. But though many physicians by this time owned automobiles, which could increase the number of patients a physician could visit in a day, it seems that not every physician was willing to travel all over the city to oversee a delivery.[19] More active physicians as well as those practitioners who took only a case or two a month continued to attend births in their own neighborhoods.[20] Of 202 physicians whose addresses could be verified, 119 (about 59 percent) remained based in a district comprising between six and eight contiguous city wards.

Furthermore, the obstetrical practices of those physicians who did cross the city were no larger than those who stayed closer to home, a point underscored by the busy physician locality index of 1.45.[21] Dr. Herbert D. Sykes, for example, had an office and home in the northeast eighteenth ward. Though he delivered an average of only 2.66 babies a month, some of his women patients came from as far away as Milwaukee's southwest fourteenth ward. But all nine of the births attended by Joseph Dries in the three sampled months of 1920 were for families who lived near his South Side eleventh ward.

Specializing in Obstetrics: Neighborhood Doctors and Institutional Physicians

By the early twentieth century, physicians were replacing midwives even in urban birthing rooms, and most of these doctors were general practitioners. Nevertheless, as early as 1905, a few Milwaukee doctors began to specialize in obstetrics, and by 1920, there was a recognizable group of obstetrical specialists in the city. But though some scholars have characterized the evolution of specialists and medical specialties in America through the growth of occupational structures and institutions, not every Milwaukee obstetrical specialist followed this route.[22] Instead, some Milwaukee doctors built obstetrical practices in a way that seemed to be based on the more traditional nineteenth-century ideal of professionalism, one in which the physician had drawn authority from his or her knowledge of the community.[23]

Though most doctors in the four counties in this study oversaw an average of 1.33 deliveries per month, twenty-one Milwaukee physicians delivered an average of at least ten babies per month, a number that even in the late twentieth century defines a specialty practice in obstetrics.[24] Beginning in 1905, when four Milwaukee physicians could be identified as concentrating in obstetrics, the number of physicians in the city with large obstetrical practices grew slowly. In 1910, four doctors in the sample fit this description, but by 1915, the number had grown to eleven, and by 1920, there were thirteen (see Table 7.1).

What factors led to the emergence of these physicians as obstetrical specialists? Throughout the nineteenth century, most American doctors were highly suspicious of the claims of medical specialists. In-

Table 7.1   Milwaukee physicians handling ten or more births per month, by year

Year	Physician	Mean no. of births per month	Declared specialty
1905	J. A. Birkl	10.33	none
	E. J. Purtell	12.33	none
	C. H. Lewis	14.00	none
	J. N. Rock	17.33	none
1910	E. J. Purtell	10.00	none
	J. A. Birkl	12.67	none
	K. Wagner	21.67	none
	F. S. Wasielewski	36.00	none
1915	P. G. Haukwitz	10.00	none
	Lam. Hargarten	10.67	Obstetrics
	J. A. Birkl	12.33	none
	W. C. Maas	13.33	none
	F. S. Wasielewski	13.67	none
	S. L. Krzysko	14.33	none
	E. J. Purtell	14.33	Surgery
	N. W. Hollenbeck	15.00	Obstetrics
	A. J. Muckerheide	15.67	Obstetrics
	A. A. Krygier	22.00	Obstetrics
	K. Wagner	22.67	none
1920	E. J. Purtell	10.33	Surgery
	Aug. Doer	10.33	none
	O. L. Bergner	11.00	none
	Lam. Hargarten	11.33	Obstetrics
	G. A. Hipke	11.33	Ob-gyn
	F. C. Liefert	11.33	not listed
	A. J. Muckerheide	12.00	Obstetrics
	J. C. Schroeder	13.33	none
	R. W. Roethke	17.00	Prof. obstet.
	N. W. Hollenbeck	17.33	Obstetrics
	S. A. Baranowski	17.67	none
	F. S. Wasielewski	18.33	none
	S. L. Krzysko	19.67	none

Sources: Data on declared specialty from Polk's *Medical and Surgical Register of the U.S.* (Detroit: R.L. Polk, 1906); American Medical Association, *American Medical Directory* (Chicago: American Medical Association, 1916, 1921).

Note: All those declaring an obstetrical specialty declared that their practice was not limited to that specialty.

deed, one Milwaukee doctor later recalled that when he began his practice in the city in 1897, the term " 'specialist' carried a subtle odium," due to the "uncontrolled reprehensible advertising of quack venereal and hernia practitioners, who invariably announced themselves to be 'specialists.' "[25] As late as the 1920s, L. H. Pelton, a past president of the Wisconsin Medical Society, argued that those medical graduates who took up specialties directly after graduation were untrustworthy. Countering the claims of a Maryland physician who had denigrated country doctors, Dr. Pelton claimed that "safe, careful, conservative" specialists needed "at least ten years in general practice," preferably in a "country practice where one has to be thrown on his own resources. They learn to make use of that which is at hand, and not to rely entirely on machine made thought and appliances."[26]

Dr. Pelton's definition of specialists as urban practitioners dependent upon machines and appliances is the most common characterization of the development of specialism. As a number of historians and sociologists have argued, American medicine in the early decades of the twentieth century became dominated by scientists and researchers. These academic doctors, invested with the increasing power and influence of the research laboratory, pushed the profession and the practice of medicine towards specialization. The growth of hospitals and other medical institutions also have been seen as a key development in promoting specialism. Aided by advances in bacteriology, which enabled the rapid growth of surgical practice in this period, some surgeons began to move their practice and even their middle-class patients to hospitals.[27] As Charles E. Rosenberg has shown, the growth of specialty outpatient clinics and later of specialty inpatient wards paralleled a gradual acceptance of the technical superiority of specialty practice, at least within the hospital.[28]

But given the focus of educational reform in Wisconsin as described in Chapter 5, perhaps it is not surprising that few of these institutional or academic factors could be used to predict the movement towards specialization taken by the Milwaukee doctors listed in Table 7.1. With an average date of graduation from medical school of 1902, the medical education and proclaimed styles of practice of these doctors were little different from those of the doctors who had similar graduation dates but small obstetrical practices: all but one of the twenty-one physicians were "regular" physicians, and only Karl

Wagner had a foreign medical degree. All of these doctors described themselves on their licenses as being in "general practice," and even a declared interest in obstetrics did not correspond with a certain level of activity. Although five of these physicians indicated in the 1921 AMA *American Medical Directory* that they were interested in obstetrics, none of them limited their practice solely to obstetrics. Indeed, the three physicians with the highest totals in 1920 did not report their concentration in obstetrics or any other specialty.[29] Institutional affiliations also were not a key to identifying obstetrical specialists: not one of the thirteen physicians in 1920 belonged to any specialty society concerned with obstetrics or obstetrics and gynecology, and only Drs. Roethke and Hipke were involved in academic obstetrics.[30] On the other hand, Dr. Wasielewski, one of the most active doctors in the group, had acted as an instructor to several of the city's midwives, taking them on as apprentices.[31]

Though hospital practice by physicians in the early twentieth century has been seen as an important indicator of specialty development, hospital practice was not an important determinant of the number of maternity cases assumed by Milwaukee's obstetricians.[32] This should not be entirely surprising, given the analysis of physician education in Chapter 5. Unlike many of the hospital physicians in the large East Coast cities in this period, doctors in Milwaukee who began to specialize early in the twentieth century had little postgraduate hospital experience.[33] In fact, though there were at least five hospitals in Milwaukee by 1915 that accepted maternity cases, only four of the eleven obstetricians identified in 1915 as having a large practice indicative of specialization were listed as being on the obstetrical staff of a hospital. Indeed, the vast majority of the thirty-four physicians who were listed as obstetrical staff physicians for these hospitals were *not* physicians with large maternity practices.[34]

The lack of a strong association in Milwaukee between physicians with large obstetrical practices and the usual standards for defining specialists illuminates the larger problem of historical context in defining "professionals" and "specialists" in the early twentieth century. Physicians themselves employed multiple criteria in claiming obstetrical specialism in this period and, as shown above, institutional or academic affiliation did not necessarily correlate with patterns of work. Indeed, not one of the seven Milwaukee doctors in 1900 listed in one medical directory as obstetrical specialists delivered significant numbers of babies that year, and only seven of the twenty-nine physicians listed in a 1921 directory delivered more than ten babies per month.[35]

These multiple meanings of specialism in the early twentieth century help to explain why the move from midwife to physician-attended childbirth depended as much on the social characteristics of the physician as on his or her medical credentials. Whatever the changes in the epistemological underpinning of medicine,[36] patients in the early years of the twentieth century continued to choose their healer within an older context based on shared cultural ideas. Midwifery attendance was one of the important cultural components of a traditional childbirth, but as Judith Walzer Leavitt has argued, the change to physician-assisted childbirth did not signify the end of all the aspects of traditional "social" childbirth. Women accepted science, Leavitt argues, but on their own terms, and they negotiated with their doctors for what they considered appropriate treatment.[37] Furthermore, despite the ascendance of the laboratory in this period, the problem for obstetrics, as noted earlier by Dr. Newman, was that other than its helping physicians understand the connection between bacteria and puerperal fever, the laboratory provided no direct link to practice. Critics could, and did, point to deficiencies of medical school training in obstetrics, but these problems could be remedied by more experience with patients at the bedside. Thus, the growth of obstetrics as a medical specialty did not necessarily rely on an institution. While some doctors would call for moving childbirth to the hospital, others found that they could build an obstetrical specialty practice in a more traditional way, by calling on their close neighborhood and ethnic ties.[38] The concept of the expert professional owed a great deal to the ethnic bonds between doctor and patient. The biography of Dr. Frank Wasielewski illustrates the particular relationship between some doctors' professional development as physicians and their membership in the community.

The son of Polish immigrant parents, Frank Wasielewski was born in Bay City, Michigan. After finishing his medical training at the University of Michigan in 1899, he settled in Milwaukee's South Side Polish community, and in 1904 he married the daughter of a prominent Milwaukee Polish immigrant family. From the beginning of his practice, he was interested in obstetrics in his community. As noted in Chapter 1, Dr. Wasielewski helped to train several Polish mid-wives.[39] At the same time, he concentrated his own practice in obstetrics; in 1905 he attended 29 births in a three-month period. Throughout the next three decades, he continued an active maternity practice; indeed, in three months in 1910 he attended 108 births, though by 1920 the three-month total had dropped to 55.

With the number of his obstetrical patients per month exceeding even late twentieth-century standards, Dr. Wasielewski moved his practice towards a specialization in obstetrics. However, like the patients of older physicians and midwives, the demographic characteristics of his patients (summarized in Table 7.2) reflected the ethnic and class structure of this neighborhood: in 1910 and 1915, less than a quarter of his patients were American-born; even in 1920, less than half of his patients were American-born, the rest having been born in Poland, the wives of artisans and laborers.[40] The geographic measures of his practice showed a similar picture: though his locality index exceeded one, all of his patients came from the South Side wards near his own fifth ward.

Within the group of twenty-one active obstetricians, four other physicians, Karl Wagner, S. L. Krzysko, A. A. Krygier, and S. A. Baranowski, were similar in many ways to Dr. Wasielewski. Except for Karl Wagner, who had trained in Germany, all had received an American medical degree, and the percentage of American-born patients for all of these doctors remained well below the mean for all doctors doing obstetrics in these years. Like Dr. Wasielewski, these four doctors lived on Milwaukee's South Side, and their locality indices show that the geographic dimensions of their obstetrical practice remained within their community (see Table 7.2).

These South Side physicians, however, were not isolated practitioners within the Polish immigrant community. Unlike some other American cities, where Italian and Slavic doctors were almost unrepresented in hospitals, Wasielewski and other Milwaukee physicians of Polish background did gain some acceptance into the city's medical establishment.[41] In 1911, for example, Drs. Wasielewski and Wagner were among those South Side physicians recruited by the reform-minded Child Welfare Commission to staff a demonstration baby clinic for poor families.[42] By 1914, Wasielewski was serving as presi-

Specializing Obstetrics

Table 7.2 Milwaukee large-practice obstetricians: Ethnicity and location of practice

Year	Physician	Locality index	Doctor birthplace	Parent birthplace	% American patients
1905	J. A. Birkl	0.826	Wis.	Ger.	58.1
	E. J. Purtell	1.882	Wis.	Can.	86.5
	C. H. Lewis	0.963	U.S.	U.S.	53.7
	J. N. Rock	1.514	Wis.	Ger.	30.8
	Mean all doctors				68.5
1910	E. J. Purtell	2.132	Wis.	Can.	62.1
	J. A. Birkl	1.445	Wis.	Ger.	73.7
	K. Wagner	1.795	Pol.	Pol.	21.3
	F. S. Wasielewski	1.821	U.S.	Pol.	23.1
	Mean all doctors				67.7
1915	P. G. Haukwitz	0.593	Ger.	Ger.	56.7
	Lam. Hargarten	0.633	Ger.	Ger.	65.6
	J. A. Birkl	1.297	Wis.	Ger.	81.1
	W. C. Maas	1.100	Wis.	—	42.1
	F. S. Wasielewski	1.816	U.S.	Pol.	22.0
	S. L. Krzysko	1.143	—	Pol.	20.9
	E. J. Purtell	1.357	Wis.	Can.	55.8
	N. W. Hollenbeck	0.641	Wis.	U.S.	75.6
	A. J. Muckerheide	1.000	Wis.	Ger.	85.1
	A. A. Krygier	1.470	U.S.	Pol.	30.8
	K. Wagner	1.537	Pol.	Pol.	35.3
	Mean all doctors				69.3
1920	E. J. Purtell	1.932	Wis.	Can.	56.7
	Aug. Doer	1.394	Wis.	Ger.	54.8
	O. L. Bergner	1.065	Wis.	—	78.8
	Lam. Hargarten	1.153	Ger.	Ger.	70.6
	G. A. Hipke	2.419	Wis.	—	81.3
	F. C. Liefert	4.000	Wis.	—	79.4
	A. J. Muckerheide	1.748	Wis.	Ger.	88.9
	J. C. Schroeder	1.835	—	—	77.5
	R. W. Roethke	2.613	Wis.	Ger.	80.0
	N. W. Hollenbeck	1.660	Wis.	U.S.	75.6
	S. A. Baranowski	1.294	U.S.	Pol.	56.6
	F. S. Wasielewski	0.983	U.S.	Pol.	49.1
	S. L. Krzysko	0.931	—	Pol.	37.3
	Mean all doctors				74.2

Sources: Birth Records, Milwaukee County, 1872–1920, Vital Records Office, Wisconsin Department of Health and Human Services, Madison, Wisconsin (WDHHS); also 1870, 1880, 1900, 1910 United States and 1905 Wisconsin State Census, Manuscript Schedules for Milwaukee County.

143

dent of the board of Johnston Emergency Hospital and, like Dr. Wagner, he was listed as a member of the obstetrical staff of Misericordia Hospital.[43] But many of Wasielewski's professional loyalties also seemed to lie with his family and community: he served as president of the Grunwald Foundation, an educational organization, and president of the Pulaski Council, a group that helped to coordinate all of the various Polish organizations in Milwaukee. But Wasielewski and Wagner's organization of the Polish Physicians' and Dentists' Association best demonstrates these doctors' professional commitment to their ethnic communities. Formed in 1913, the organization seems to have been primarily a Milwaukee group, though it was described as national. Meetings were irregular at first, but within a few years, the society had grown and began to meet regularly and to present scientific papers. But the ties to the community remained strong. In 1932, the wives of association members, under the direction of Mrs. Frank Wasielewski, formed an auxiliary. Auxiliary members promoted the association, but they also reached out to the community, aiding veterans and raising money for a local orphanage.[44]

With his home delivery practice based in his own neighborhood, Wasielewski and the other doctors in the immigrant Polish community were pivotal figures in the adaptation of social childbirth from midwife- to physician-assisted. When they began their practice, these doctors worked with midwives even as they added obstetrics cases to their own practices.[45] As active members of the Polish community, these doctors combined an understanding of Polish cultural values with their knowledge of the possibilities of scientific medicine. Thus, as birthing women on Milwaukee's South Side began to demand professional birth attendants, they called on the "professionals" who were recognized in their community. Though these doctors represented a change in gender in the birthing room, their ethnic ties provided a strong link with tradition. One demonstration of this link is shown by the location of the births. Though some physicians in the city were moving their deliveries to the hospital, all five of these doctors attended births almost solely at home.[46]

In assuming some of the largest caseloads of any of the doctors in this study, Dr. Wasielewski and the other doctors in Milwaukee's Polish community built specialist practices that relied more on the traditional face-to-face expectations of the nineteenth-century doctor-patient relationship.[47] But the evolution of medical institutions in the city and in the state by the second decade of the twentieth century facilitated the development of another type of obstetrical specialist. These specialists would define themselves by their institutional and academic affiliations, not by their cultural ties. Indeed, even the number of obstetrical cases they oversaw sometimes seemed irrelevant.[48]

The Wisconsin State Medical Society offered one of the first forums for physicians who wished to stake a public claim for obstetric specialization. Though Milwaukee physicians, such as Dr. Alois Graettinger, tended to dominate the society's Committee on Obstetrics, Dr. Julius Noer, a Stoughton (Dane County) physician, became chairman in 1900. Though Noer was unwilling to excoriate midwives, he was an outspoken advocate of the "necessity of proper and scientific handling of these [obstetrical] cases." Though he practiced in a small town, he was also an early promoter of hospitalization for maternity cases. In 1906, he argued that "all confinement cases should be placed in a lying-in hospital . . . where women will be properly, aseptically and scientifically cared for during and after labor. Every municipality should be required by law to maintain a properly equipped lying-in hospital."[49]

Though the medical schools in Milwaukee had been founded as profit-making ventures, by the early twentieth century they provided an institutional affiliation for their professors who understood and desired the prestige value of these links.[50] For doctors like Gustav Hipke, who were interested in obstetrics, a medical school post affirmed their commitment to the subject. Hipke had been a country doctor in Kiel, Wisconsin, until 1899, when he went to Chicago for two years to study obstetrics. In 1901, he and his wife moved to Milwaukee, and by 1904, he was Professor of Obstetrics at the Wisconsin College of Physicians and Surgeons.[51] By 1906, with the aid of his wife Clara, Hipke had founded the Milwaukee Maternity Hospital "for needy mothers and their babies."[52]

But like the eight other doctors in this study between 1900 and 1920 who claimed a medical school post in obstetrics, Hipke was not a particularly active obstetrician. In 1905, for example, Hipke attended only one delivery in three months; and Byron Nobles, Professor of Obstetrics at the Milwaukee Medical College, delivered an average of 5.67 babies per month, the most of the four academic obstetricians in practice in this year.[53] By 1915, when Marquette University had taken over medical education in Milwaukee, the three obstetrical professors averaged only 2.44 births per month.[54] Only Rudolph Roethke, who was an obstetrics professor at Marquette in 1920, attended a substantial number of births (mean of 16.67 per month in 1920).

Though Roethke and Hipke had relatively large obstetrical practices by 1920, they were representative of a new type of obstetrical practitioner who evaluated specialism more in terms of its relationship with particular institutions than with the actual number of patients they oversaw. The American Medical Association's *Medical Directory* provided one such institutional link. By 1921 in the four counties of this study, thirty-four physicians claimed to be obstetrical specialists in the AMA *Directory*. Though the *Directory* cautioned that these claims to specialty practice were purely self-defined and therefore not verifiable, they still represented a conscious decision by a physician to claim the status of a specialist.[55] But, like the academic obstetricians, there was little relationship between this claim to specialization and the actual size of an obstetrician's practice. While the average number of births all the doctors in Milwaukee in this study in 1920 was 2.4 per month, for the twenty-nine self-described obstetrical specialists in Milwaukee, the average number of births per month was 5.3, still far less than that of the thirteen large practice doctors of 1920 described above, who averaged 13.9 deliveries per month.[56]

However, the twenty-nine practitioners in this group were distinguishable by two factors that were part of the professionalizing process of specialty practice in the twentieth century: the nationality of their patients and their use of the hospital. While the thirteen large practice doctors had historically delivered a substantial number of immigrant women, those AMA specialists in practice as early as 1905 attended predominantly American-born women. As Table 7.3 shows, these doctors did not practice in the Polish community, and only a few of their patients came from Milwaukee's German community.[57] In addition to the high percentages of American patients, unlike many physicians in the city, these doctors were more likely to attend a birth in a hospital. In 1920, 78.4 percent of the births attended by all the physicians in the study took place at home. While the large practice

Table 7.3 Types of obstetrical specialists: Ethnicity of patients of large practice obstetricians vs. AMA-advertised obstetricians, 1905–1920

Year	Type of doctor	Mean % of obstetrical patients		
		American	German	Polish
1905	All doctors	66.0	19.7	3.5
	Large practice	51.8	23.2	13.6
	AMA-defined	82.8	13.6	3.6
1910	All doctors	67.7	17.8	2.0
	Large practice	56.4	19.9	14.0
	AMA-defined	56.7	14.2	5.6
1915	All doctors	69.3	12.3	3.6
	Large practice	60.0	11.2	16.1
	AMA-defined	64.4	10.9	4.1
1920	All doctors	74.0	5.5	4.5
	Large practice	66.9	5.2	15.0
	AMA-defined	72.8	4.8	6.9

Sources: Birth Records, Milwaukee County (1905, 1910, 1915, 1920), WDHHS; also American Medical Association, *American Medical Directory* (Chicago: American Medical Association, 1921), pp. 1597–1603.

physicians, who averaged between 14 and 15 births per month, hospitalized only 17.9 percent of their obstetrical cases, the physicians who claimed obstetrical specialization in the AMA *Directory* and averaged about 5 births per month, hospitalized 42.9 percent of their maternity patients.[58]

Though many doctors in this time period cited the advantages of the hospital for maternity cases in rather vague terms as "cleaner" or "more scientific," some obstetricians, such as Rudolph Roethke, found the hospital to be a place to advance the scientific qualities of obstetrical practice.[59] Indeed, the story of Dr. Roethke illustrates the significant cultural differences between the neighborhood obstetricians and those who came to dominate medical practice in the twentieth century. Born in Wisconsin, Dr. Roethke attended the University of Wisconsin for several years before he went to medical school at the University of Pennsylvania. After his graduation in 1910, he spent a year as an intern and ten additional months as a house surgeon at the New York Lying-In Hospital. In 1912, he moved to Milwaukee and opened an office practice in a fashionable downtown building.

For the first five years of his practice, he delivered babies as part of a general practice, but in 1917, he decided to specialize in obstetrics. By 1920, he was a Professor of Obstetrics at Marquette University Medical School and on the staff of three other Milwaukee hospitals.[60] Dr. Roethke's patients came from a significantly different community of Milwaukee than the patients who consulted Dr. Wasielewski and the other Polish physicians.[61] For the three sampled months of 1920, over 80 percent of Roethke's patients were born in the United States and 58 percent of them were from white-collar families. Only 2 percent of his patients were the wives of laborers.[62] Furthermore, almost all of his deliveries took place in hospitals.

With his postgraduate training in obstetrics, an academic post as Professor of Obstetrics, and his practice based primarily in the hospital, Dr. Roethke represented the ideal of the twentieth-century scientific specialist. Though he eventually left academic medicine to return to full-time private practice, he published a number of articles in medical journals as well as a medical students' and nurses' guide to obstetrics, and he was well known in state medical circles for his willingness to try new techniques in obstetrical surgery.[63] In fact, his enthusiasm for performing cesarean sections caused some conflict in Milwaukee medical circles. In 1918, he presented a paper before the Surgical Section of the State Medical Society entitled "Indications for Davis Caesarian Section." Reporting on thirty-three cases of cesarean section, performed usually due to several obstetric complications, Roethke argued for the increased use of these surgical deliveries. Women and babies would be saved, he argued, pointing out that his maternal mortality rate in an uncomplicated case was about 1 percent; in cases with complications, the rate was 3 to 10 percent. But while a few physicians present at the talk supported Roethke's surgical prowess, with one physician noting that he had helped Roethke perform many of the reported operations, others were more critical. For example, Dr. P. H. McGovern, a Milwaukee practitioner, reported that he had been in a Milwaukee hospital two months previously when Dr. Roethke was performing this surgery. When McGovern asked an intern about the indications for the operation, the intern told him that he did not think there were any. Roethke denied any impropriety, but the chair of the session noted at the end that "I have heard whispering from time to time in Milwaukee, and I trust this subject will come up again and again until we all see the indications and agree upon them as we should, whether the facts are all as Doctor Roethke says or not."[64]

The comparison of Dr. Wasielewski's home and ethnic-community-based specialist practice with Dr. Roethke's academic and hospital-based obstetric practice reveals the difficulties in defining a medical specialist in the early twentieth century. Furthermore, because the professionalization of obstetrics has been used as a mechanism for understanding why midwife practice disappeared in the United States, it is important to delineate the parameters of specialization in this crucial transition period. As the stories of these two doctors illustrate, there were several routes to specialist practice. While the academic model of Dr. Roethke is the one that has been used by historians to explain the disappearance of midwife practice, the home-based, ethnic practice of Dr. Wasielewski is probably the more appropriate model for understanding the change to doctor-attended childbirth. Dr. Wasielewski's patients, immigrant women who might have sought out the services of a midwife, chose him instead. Many upper- and middle-class native-born women, particularly those in urban areas, were consulting doctors for their confinements by the end of the nineteenth century. Women of this class, accustomed to physicians, by the first decades of the twentieth century were moving from general practitioners to seeking out specialists like Dr. Roethke.[65]

But while both kinds of obstetrical specialists could practice in these early years of the twentieth century, only Dr. Roethke's model would prevail. Supported by institutions that increasingly were identified as the only place to practice scientific medicine, obstetricians like Dr. Roethke would displace more community-oriented physicians like Dr. Wasielewski or Dr. Wagner. But, as many historians have shown, the institutions of scientific medicine were not culturally neutral. Hospitals in particular had always been the province of the American elite, and by the 1930s, professional organizations such as the American Board of Obstetricians and Gynecologists would claim that only specialists they approved should practice in hospitals. Established in 1930, the Board instituted a national group whose aims included putting a stamp of approval on qualified practitioners.[66] From the beginning, the Board refused to certify part-time specialists or any practitioner who accepted male patients, criteria that had the effect of delineating clear boundaries between the specialist and the general practitioner.[67] By 1936, the Board's power had extended to defining who could and could not practice in a hospital. The lay public and hospital directors, the Board claimed, had come to use certification as a "means of discriminating between those who are well grounded as specialists and those who are not."[68]

Thus, Milwaukee and other physicians who wished to specialize in obstetrics after 1930 would not find professional affiliation with such groups as the German physicians' group Verein Deutscher Aerzte or the Polish Physicians' and Dentists' Association.[69] Professional bonds would be forged within the medical institution, and not within the doctor's larger community. Unlike the situation in the early twentieth century, after 1930 only American medical institutions would be acceptable. By the 1940s, in fact, the Wisconsin Board of Medical Examiners refused to license a number of foreign medical graduates who were displaced persons, claiming that a Ph.D. and an M.D. from foreign schools were not as good as the training "our own boys" received.[70]

Birthing women followed their doctors to the accepted institutions, and by the 1930s, despite the terrible economic toll of the Great Depression, well over half of births in urban areas took place in hospitals.[71] But, as Rosemary Stevens has shown, the very organization of the twentieth-century hospital worked against doctors forging relationships with the hospital staff, and this lack of cohesiveness led to the depersonalization of hospital care.[72]

By the 1950s and 1960s, birthing women began to protest this type of hospital care, arguing that though scientific medicine offered safety and health, it was also inhumane and insensitive. Even more alarming was the growing evidence that this model of American maternity care was not preventing death. Referring to the rather dismal American infant mortality statistics relative to the rest of the developed world, critics pointed out that the United States ranked well below the top ten countries with the lowest mortality rates; in one study, the United States ranked sixteenth, below such places as Hong Kong.[73] While social and economic factors were partly to blame, some studies suggested that the institutional model itself was at fault. Indeed, the American College of Obstetricians and Gynecologists' own research revealed that the larger the obstetric service and the stronger the affiliation between an obstetric service and a medical school, the greater the rate of infant and maternal deaths.[74] The time had come, many believed, for a reconsideration of the cultural and social aspects of childbirth.

Gender, Ethnicity, and the Meanings of Professionalism

On May 15, 1915, Anna Rosina Zoladkiewicz, a Polish-American woman living in Milwaukee, Wisconsin, called Dr. Frank Wasielewski to deliver her tenth child. Like Dr. Wasielewski, Mrs. Zoladkiewicz lived in Milwaukee's South Side, a predominantly working-class and ethnically Polish neighborhood. Her economic and social circumstances were typical of her community. But what makes her confinement interesting is Mrs. Zoladkiewicz herself. A thirty-eight-year-old school-educated midwife who was an active practitioner in the community, Mrs. Zoladkiewicz shared an occupational interest in childbirth with her physician. However, as this was to be only her fourth living baby out of ten deliveries, perhaps her desire to ensure a safe outcome led her to decide to call in a physician attendant for this birth.[1]

This example of a Milwaukee midwife hiring a local physician to attend her own confinement in the early years of the twentieth century illustrates two important aspects of this study of the professionalization of childbirth in the late nineteenth and early twentieth centuries, namely gender and culture. Her choice of a physician for this birth demonstrates the conflict between gender and professionalization. Though Mrs. Zoladkiewicz was one of many trained midwives living on Milwaukee's South Side, she hired a physician—a professional male—from her community when she needed help for her own delivery. Her choice of a male doctor was ordained by circumstances: though there were several women physicians in Milwaukee, not one had indicated an interest in obstetrics. Indeed, there was no female specialist in obstetrics in Milwaukee until 1950.[2] Mrs. Zoladkiewicz's particular choice of Dr. Wasielewski points out the second major issue of this study. Mrs. Zoladkiewicz turned to a professional, a physician, but one from her own community. Dr. Wasielewski was a highly respected representative of scientific medicine in Milwaukee's South Side and one of several doctors in the neighborhood who had concentrated his practice in obstetrics.[3] She and Dr. Wasielewski shared the same ethnic background, and they both lived and practiced in the same neighborhood.

Like Anna Zoladkiewicz, in the years after 1920, women in Milwaukee and the other three Wisconsin counties in this study turned increasingly to physicians to deliver their babies, and midwives were left with a very limited number of patients. In the two all-rural counties of this study, only a few midwives remained in practice after 1920. In Trempealeau County, there were only nine midwife-attended births in six months in 1920, while in Price County, seven midwives continued to attend a few births per year among the women in the Finnish community through 1930.[4] More midwives remained in practice in the urban areas of Wisconsin, as evidenced in the advertisements in the city directories. (Though the number of midwives advertising in the city directories is only a rough guide to ascertaining the number of midwives in practice, it does identify women who still sought public recognition of their services.) In Madison, there were no midwife listings in the city directories after 1919.[5] In Milwaukee, as Table C.1 illustrates, eighty-seven midwives advertised in the city directory in 1919, but after 1931, fewer than ten midwives were active in the city.

Table C.1 Midwives in Milwaukee city directories, 1919–1950

Date	No. of total midwives	No. of new midwives
1919	87	21
1925	22	2
1931	16	4
1935	8	2
1940	5	1
1945	3	0
1950	4	0

Sources: "Midwives," classified advertising section of Wright's *Milwaukee City Directory* (Milwaukee: Wright's Directory Co., 1919, 1925, 1931, 1935, 1940, 1945, 1950).

Though a few midwives still continued to work in Milwaukee even as late as 1950 (Mrs. Zoladkiewicz, for example, advertised in the city directory until 1945) the dramatic reduction in the number of midwives after 1919 bespeaks a significantly diminished call for their services.

With fewer women calling upon midwives, only a handful of women took up this occupation. Like their nineteenth-century colleagues, all of these twentieth-century urban midwives were immigrants who wanted to serve women within their own ethnic communities. Thus, it was not surprising when three midwives in 1924 petitioned the Committee on Midwives of the State Medical Practice Board to give the licensure examinations in Polish, Italian, and German.[6] At another meeting in 1922, Board member Dr. G. H. Ripley argued on behalf of Rosa Cesario, who wanted to practice in his hometown of Kenosha. Noting that "this midwife is needed in the Italian colony at Kenosha," Ripley asked that the Board consider the provisions of the law as "liberally constructed" so that Cesario could receive her license.[7]

Rosa Cesario was one of the few midwives who began midwifery practice in Wisconsin in the 1920s. As Table C.1 shows, only nine new names appeared in the Milwaukee city directory listings after 1919, and no new midwives advertised after 1940. The dates midwives applied for state licenses show a similar trend. Most of the 373 midwives who registered with the state had done so in the first few years after the passage of the registration law in 1909; only 12 women registered for licenses between 1920 and 1930. In fact, by 1935, the Wisconsin State Medical Practice Board's Committee on Midwifery was combined with its committees on Chiropody and Massage. It obviously had little to do: only one midwife, Mary Cardinal, was granted a license after 1930, while two other women were turned down "due to insufficient credentials."[8]

With very few women applying for midwifery licenses by the 1930s, the physicians on the Board turned their attention to what midwives were practicing. From the beginning of the twentieth century, some physician critics of midwives had charged that immigrant midwives were often guilty of providing abortions.[9] Though at least eleven doctors and only three registered midwives in Wisconsin were convicted of performing abortions between 1923 and 1939, the Board dealt much more harshly with the midwives. In any case where a midwife was convicted of performing an "illegal operation," her registration was revoked, permanently.[10] But seven of the eleven revoked physician licenses were eventually reinstated, including those of two of the four doctors who served prison sentences for manslaughter. Political connections obviously helped: one of the two doctors, F. A. Walters, was a former mayor of Stevens Point. Though he was tried and found guilty of manslaughter of a woman in 1928, he was pardoned by the governor of Wisconsin in 1931, and his license was restored.[11]

The different punishment for physicians and midwives convicted of performing abortions reflected the established belief by the 1930s in the authority and status of professionals. The Board's investigation and prosecution of a Milwaukee midwife for the practice of "Polish medicine" in 1932 further demonstrates the gender and cultural distance between this professional world and the one where immigrant midwives lived. Josephine Krzyzanowska had trained in midwifery at a Chicago school after her arrival from Poland in 1892. She registered with the city of Milwaukee in 1907 and with the state in 1910. Though she attended only a few births, like many traditional midwives, she was called on to diagnose and treat minor illnesses among many members of her community. However, while many midwives in traditional societies prescribed medicines as well as birthed babies, Josephine Krzyzanowska's practice of this type of traditional medicine well into the twentieth century was unusual, and it attracted the attention of the State Board of Medical Examiners. They began their investigation by attempting to persuade people within the community to testify against her. However, the community refused. As Walter Drews, the exasperated medical investigator, explained, "This was a case similar to many others involving the practicing of Polish medicine women, where testimony against the offender was impossible to secure by bona fide patients." The state examiner then sent two female deputies to entrap Krzyzanowska, who was arrested and charged with practicing medicine without a license.[12]

Though many within the Milwaukee's Polish community were reluctant to help the Board of Medical Examiners prosecute Krzyzanowska, they increasingly forsook midwifery services like hers to call upon physician birth attendants based within their community.[13] But the changeover from physicians to board-certified specialists was slow in Wisconsin. Though by 1940, more than fifty physicians in the four counties of this study indicated that they were specialists in obstetrics and gynecology, the number of Board-certified specialists remained low. Only eight doctors in Milwaukee and three in Madison were listed as certified specialists in a 1939 directory, and in 1950, the numbers were twenty-one in Milwaukee and four in Madison. Only two of these doctors were female.[14]

But though there were relatively few certified obstetrical specialists, the practice of obstetrics for most Wisconsin doctors after 1920 became hospital based. In Madison, over 65 percent of the births took place in hospitals as early as 1924; by 1938, 73.2 percent of urban women in the state had hospital deliveries, a figure that approximated the national average in 1940.[15] In rural areas of the state, where hospital beds were scarce in the early twentieth century, the number of hospital births lagged behind those in the city. By the 1920s, however, many rural communities, supported by philanthropic agencies, began to build hospitals that were assumed to be centers for medical technique and symbols of community innovation and strength.[16] Small communities, such as Whitehall in Trempealeau County and Phillips in Price County, built small cottage hospitals, and they attracted parturient women: in 1940, there were at least 228 hospitals in the state and just over one-half (51.1 percent) of births in rural Wisconsin took place in these institutions, a figure that exceeded the national average of 32.3 percent.[17]

In 1916, the well-known Chicago obstetrician Joseph B. DeLee called for the elimination of midwives and the establishment of what he termed a "single standard" of obstetrics. Doing away with midwives, he argued, would establish "high ideals" for obstetrical care for all women, the well-off as well as the poor.[18] In a subsequent paper in 1920, DeLee outlined his "prophylactic forceps" procedure, a method of managing childbirth that required significant amounts of surgical and drug intervention and that had to be done in the hospital. Women's lives and reproductive functions would be preserved, he argued, and millions of babies would not grow up with debilitating head injuries.[19] By 1950, with the federal government contributing to the cost of building hospitals, most white women in the United States received obstetrical care that approximated DeLee's "ideal obstetrics." In that year, 92.8 percent of births to white mothers took place in hospitals; by 1960, the figure was close to 100 percent. The differences between urban and rural white women diminished in this time period as well: in 1940, only 36.6 percent of white rural women had hospital births, as opposed to 78.6 percent of urban white women, but in 1950, the figures were 97.1 percent and 86.0, respectively.[20]

Yet, while DeLee had struggled to include poor immigrant women in his 1916 definition of "ideal obstetrics," African-American women were never mentioned. The result was the continuation of a double standard of obstetrics tied to a very gendered and culturally defined professional ideal. The standards of scientific, male professionalism were presumed to be absolutely essential for white women, but a black female midwife, properly supervised by the state, was considered adequate for black women.[21] As late as 1940, nearly half of the babies of all nonwhite American women and 71.1 percent of rural nonwhite women were delivered by a midwife. In 1950, midwives still attended 27.8 percent of all minority women and 50.2 percent of rural nonwhite Americans. The figures for hospital births for black and other minority women were also low: in 1940, 26.7 percent of births to all nonwhite women and only 8.6 percent of births to rural minority women took place in a hospital. By 1950, though 57.9 percent of all nonwhite women went to the hospital to deliver a baby, only 30.0 percent of rural nonwhite women received this kind of obstetrical care.[22] In 1960, the numbers for black women began to approximate those of white women: 85 percent of black women in 1960 had hospital births. However, in Alabama and Mississippi, at least 40 percent of births to black women were still handled by midwives in 1960, and as late as 1970, the figures on midwife-attended births for nonwhite women in both states was still greater than 10 percent.[23] Ironically, the move to the hospital did little to lower the astonishingly high rates of infant mortality in these states: after midwives were banned in Alabama in the mid-1970s, the infant mortality rate for black babies in these states remained the highest in the country.[24]

For African-American women, the choice between a traditional birth with a midwife and DeLee's "ideal obstetrics" was restricted by racism, legal segregation, and economics.[25] But as early as the 1940s, white women were beginning to question the prevailing model of a fully drugged, physician-controlled, delivery. Yet, as several authors have argued, the methods outlined in Grantly Dick-Read's *Childbirth without Fear: The Principles and Practice of Natural Childbirth* and later in Fernand Lamaze's *Painless Childbirth* were really only intended to reform childbirth practices within the hospital.[26] By the late 1960s, however, women in the feminist movement and in the counterculture helped to kindle a reexamination of the professional model inherent in American obstetrics. While most changes occurred within the prevailing system, as women used their clout as consumers to force physicians and hospitals to change their obstetrical practices, some critics argued that the entire model needed to be discarded. Feminists such as Suzanne Arms were joined by utopian women like Ina May Gaskin in advocating a return to home birth monitored by a female midwife. This model of childbirth, they argued, supported birthing women instead of dominating them, as would happen in a hospital.[27]

Though a hospital birth directed by a physician remains the American way of birth at the end of the twentieth century, there have been changes since that standard was established. Since the early 1970s, medical schools, pushed by legal challenges to sexist admissions policies, have graduated increasing numbers of women. Many of these women have chosen to specialize in obstetrics and gynecology; the American College of Obstetricians and Gynecologists recently reported that almost 20 percent of its "Fellows" are women and that the number of women in its residency programs was approaching 50 percent.[28] To deal with the large numbers of American communities remaining drastically underserved by medical care, the medical profession also has attempted to recruit medical students from communities other than the white middle class. But the criticism of the role of the professional in providing maternity care has extended to a general critique of the narrow focus and the high cost of specialist care in hospitals. Medical schools and postgraduate training programs are now under pressure to turn out fewer specialists and train more primary- and general-care providers. Some have even suggested that expensive specialists, such as those in the surgical specialties, could be replaced with less expensive personnel.[29] Nurse-midwives, who work primarily in hospitals under the aegis of a physician, have been seen as one solution to the perceived problems of cost and the lack of individual care for parturient women.[30] Whether medical personnel can move away from their links with institutions remains to be seen, but the concerns that have been raised in recent years demonstrate that the problem of defining the relationship of professionalism, culture, and gender remains as much an issue at the end of the twentieth century as it was at the beginning.

Appendix:
Quantitative Sources

Six different data sets were used in this study of the change from midwife- to physician-assisted childbirth in Wisconsin. The Milwaukee Health Department's register of midwives (the "Physicians' Register"), the state midwife license files, the federal and state manuscript census schedules from 1870, 1880, 1900, 1905, and 1910, the Milwaukee City Directory, the state physicians' licenses, and birth certificates sampled from the four counties all provided unique information about childbirth attendants and the families who employed them. Yet, as with any study employing quantitative data, each set had particular problems and limitations. Most of my findings and the relevant statistical analyses are given in the text. This appendix describes the information, the usefulness, and the problems posed by each set. Specific uses of each data set are provided in the text.

Birth Certificates

Birth certificates filed by midwives and physicians who delivered babies provided a means of assessing individual practice and changes over time in the employment of birth attendants. Selecting four representative counties in Wisconsin, I coded records for sampled years from 1870 to 1920. A total of 28,924 birth records were coded from the records filed with the Dane County Vital Records Office in Madison and the Vital Records Office of the State of Wisconsin Department of Health and Human Services, also in Madison.

The Dane County records, which I first used in a pilot study, proved that this type of data could be useful in examining the transition from midwife- to physician-assisted childbirth. For the pilot study, I sampled the year 1870 and proceeded every five years through 1900. Due to time restrictions, 1905 births were omitted, but 1910 was coded. For this county, every birth in a given year was used, and the following variables were coded:

Month of birth
Day of birth
Year of birth
Surname of father
Parity of mother
Father's listed occupation[1]
Place of birth (area in Dane County)[2]
Mother's birthplace[3]
Father's birthplace
Complications (if listed)[4]
Attendant number (each doctor and midwife was given a code)
Attendant's home (area in Dane County)[5]
Attendant's status[6]

Because the focus of my study involved an analysis of the cultural dimensions of the change in childbirth attendants in both urban and rural Wisconsin, I designed the larger study using birth certificates from three more representative Wisconsin counties in addition to the data already collected from Dane County. The choice of an urban area was obvious: Milwaukee County included the city of Milwaukee, the largest urban area in the state. In addition, a number of historical studies have focused on industry and health in Milwaukee, and they provided a larger context for this study.[7] Merle Curti's previous work on Trempealeau County provided the context for a study of rural childbirth attendants.[8] However, Trempealeau was a settled rural county by 1870 and was not representative of many rural areas of Wisconsin. A center of the logging industry in northern Wisconsin, Price County was representative of many of the sparsely settled frontier areas in northern Wisconsin. Part of the "cut-over" timber areas in the northern part of the state, it was carved out of parts of Lincoln and Chippewa Counties and became a separate county in 1879.[9]

In deciding what periods of time and which years should be coded, several issues had to be considered. At least several months of each year needed to be coded in order to evaluate trends in midwives' or physicians' practices. In addition, part of the strategy for this study involved being able to trace practitioners to other sources, such as licenses and the manuscript census schedules. Given the vastly different numbers of birth certificates filed within each county, one scheme would not work for all counties. Thus, for Trempealeau and Milwaukee County, all the births were coded for sampled months during the years 1873, 1877, 1880, 1885, 1890, 1895, 1900, 1905, 1910, 1915, and 1920. Because the records in Price County did not start until 1880, coding began with that year and was followed by sampled months every five years, as for the two other counties. To obtain a manageable, yet representative, data set, varying numbers of months for each sampled year were coded: in Milwaukee County, four months were coded in the years 1873, 1877, and 1880,[10] but in the years between 1885 and 1920, three-month periods were used. For Trempealeau County, births were coded for an entire year in every sampled year through 1900, and for six-month periods in the four sampled years between 1905 and 1920. For Price County, births were recorded for all the sampled years between 1880 and 1905, and then for six-month periods in the years 1910, 1915, and 1920.[11]

Though the birth certificate forms changed somewhat over the years studied, I was able to code the following variables for Milwaukee, Trempealeau, and Price Counties:

County
Month of birth
Day of birth
Year of birth
Street number (for Milwaukee City only)
Street name (for Milwaukee City only; for other towns of Milwaukee County and for towns of Price and Trempealeau County, town name noted here)
Place of birth[12]
Father's occupation[13]
Father's birthplace[14]
Mother's birthplace

Parity of mother[15]
Complications[16]
Attendant number
Attendant status[17]
Hospital number (if hospital birth, which hospital)[18]
Ward number (for Milwaukee City only)

There were both advantages and problems with this data set. The sheer size of the two data sets for all four counties—over 28,000 births—and the span of time covered by the set—fifty years—permitted a detailed analysis of change over time. It allowed a study of the geographic, class, ethnic, and medical factors of childbirth practice that changed over time—details that are not available anywhere else for such a large and varied group of midwives or doctors.[19] The size of the set helped to compensate for missing variables for certain years, and it allowed for subdivision into smaller sets for more specialized study, such as groups of midwives or groups of doctors. The attendant numbers enabled me to link this file with several other files containing information on midwives and doctors. Thus, by aggregating the birth file by attendant number, it was possible to merge information about practice with the data sets on education and family.

The largest problem with this data set had to do with the population represented in this study. Though state and local statutes mandated the reporting of births, Wisconsin did not join the federally sponsored Birth Registration Area until 1917, two years after it was first established. Thus, though reporting was high, probably between 90 and 95 percent, not every birth in the state was reported, and there did not seem to be severe sanctions for non-reporting. The gap in reporting was more significant in rural than in urban areas. However, contemporary observers noted that midwives reported births as frequently as physicians did.[20] Thus, any bias in my birth sample is probably equal for both types of practitioners.[21] In addition, I was unable to code illegitimate births after 1907, due to a state law that mandated that they be separately reported and kept confidential.[22]

Other problems with the birth certificates related to how the form changed over time. Ward boundaries in Milwaukee changed, so wards could not be compared in different years. Parental birthplace was not noted until 1880, and in 1900 and 1905, parental addresses were not recorded in Milwaukee. Thus, another means of obtaining these addresses had to be devised in order to follow the geographic factors of practice. For each of the sampled births for these two years, I linked parents' names and occupations to the city directories and the manuscript census schedules in order to fill in the addresses and determine the ward where the birth took place.

Milwaukee Health Department Physicians' Register

In 1877, the city of Milwaukee Health Department began requiring that midwives practicing in the city register with the Health Department. The names of midwives who complied with this directive, as well as the names of physicians practicing in the city and the names of women who were running so-called baby farms, were entered in this registry. The Physicians' Register, which contains all three lists of names, is now located at the Milwaukee Public Library Archives.

In the thirty years between 1877 and 1907, when the Register ends, there were 658 midwife entries. However, the number of entries exceeded the number of women who actually registered. In 1906 and in 1907, some women who had registered previously with the Health Department reregistered. When duplicate entries were eliminated, the actual total of midwives was 588.

Because of the length of time covered by the Register, this data set provided a dynamic look at midwife qualifications over the thirty-year period. It also provided possible lists of the graduates of Milwaukee's two schools of midwifery. In the 1880s and 1890s, graduates of the Milwaukee School of Midwifery and the Wisconsin College of Midwifery registered in groups, often within the month that they graduated. Though most graduates were residents of the city, a few midwives recorded addresses outside of the city.

There were several problems with this source. It is unclear what measures the Health Department employed to encourage midwives to register. Though there were no specific requirements that a midwife needed to fulfill in order to be registered, midwives who attended only a few births and/or midwives who were not graduates of the Milwaukee schools are probably underrepresented. In addition, though many midwives reported school training, they provided little information beyond the name of the school and the year of graduation.

The following variables were coded from the Registry:

Date of registration—month, day, year
Midwife's last name
Midwife's first name or the first initial
Midwife's street address—street number
Midwife's street address—street name
Midwife's ward number (if reported)
Country of training[23]
College or school where midwife was trained[24]
Year of graduation
Doctor reference no. 1[25]
Doctor reference no. 2
Prime residence—where midwife's permanent home was located
    (Milwaukee or out of town)

State Midwife Licenses

In 1909, an amendment to the State Medical Practice Act of Wisconsin mandated that midwives practicing in the state of Wisconsin apply for licenses from the State of Wisconsin Board of Medical Examiners. The statute required every midwife who wished to practice in the state after 1909 to apply for a certificate of registration.[26] To be granted a certificate, a midwife had to meet three criteria: graduation from a "reputable" school of midwifery (defined as one offering a twelve-month course of instruction in a hospital or sanitarium); experience with at least twenty confinement cases; and evidence of "good moral and professional character," which amounted to recommendations from two physicians and one layperson, preferably a clergyman. In addition, the prospective midwife had to pass a written examination conducted by the Board of Medical Examiners.[27] A key provision of the statute, however, exempted midwives who had been practicing in the state prior to the passage of this bill. They did not have to meet the educational requirements, nor did they have to take the exam. Thus, any midwife already in practice received a license, regardless of her preparation to be a midwife.

A total of 373 practicing midwives applied for registration after 1909 under this statute. Most of them registered within the first few years after the passage of the statute, although one application was dated as late as 1939. Most of the midwives therefore received their licenses automatically, since they were in practice before 1909. Unlike the physician licenses (discussed below), whose forms changed over time, all of the 373 midwife license applications asked for the same information about residence, schooling, and references. The files are now kept at the Archives Division of the Wisconsin State Historical Society (Series 1611). The variables that I coded included:

Midwife's last name
Initial of first name
Marital status[28]
County
City
Street number
Street name
Age as reported
Kind of training[29]
Midwifery school attended[30]
Months of training
Year of graduation
Months of hospital work
Number of cases attended
Years practiced in Wisconsin
Years practiced in United States
Years practiced in Europe
Total number of years in practice
If European, which country
Doctor no. 1 county[31]
Doctor no. 2 county
Doctor no. 1 number[32]
Doctor no. 2 number
Layperson number[33]

These license files were a rich source of information about the level of midwife training in Wisconsin. They provided details such as the specific school, the number of months of training, and even the number of months of hospital work for each midwife. In addition, many of the women wrote extensive details about their training, perhaps in an attempt to justify their competence. Many of these comments, while not easily converted to numbers, I found useful in trying to understand how these women felt about their midwifery education. Because many of the graduates of the Milwaukee midwifery schools applied for licenses, it was possible to piece together information about the curriculum from these schools—information that does not exist anywhere else. The details provided by the registrants are probably fairly accurate, since every woman who was already practicing automatically received a license. In addition, most of the active midwives I found in other sources applied for licenses. Thus, the details provided by the midwives in the midwife license file were fairly representative of most midwives' experiences in the state.

However, the cost, though small ($5 for women already in practice), as well as the inconvenience of obtaining the form and finding physician references probably kept midwives with very small practices from bothering to register. Thus, neighbor-woman midwives may be underrepresented in the state licenses. However, these women were not invisible: most signed birth certificates regardless of their status. As noted in Chapter 3, a number of rural women delivered babies without having registered with the state, and a contemporary study of childbearing conditions in Marathon County found several unregistered midwives. These midwives, however, had very small practices.[34]

Federal and State Censuses

Midwives, usually the wives of immigrant, working-class families, did not leave the letters or diaries that have traditionally provided historians with the details of women's lives. In addition, we know very little about the circumstances of ordinary physicians. Thus, the details about midwives' and physicians' families found in the federal manuscript census schedules for 1870, 1880, 1900, and 1910 and the state of Wisconsin manuscript census schedule for 1905 proved very useful. I used the Soundex system to locate particular midwife and physician names and addresses, which I then traced to microfilm copies of the manuscript census schedules for the four counties. I was able to link 398 of a total of 893 midwives (44.6 percent) and 598 of 1,149 physicians (52.0 percent) to the various censuses. I attempted to link practitioners to the census nearest to the date when they first began to practice because I wanted to capture the full effect of family life on their practice. The following variables were coded for all censuses, though the census schedules from 1900, 1905, and 1910 provided more details than the ones from 1870 and 1880.

Census year
Midwife or doctor number (each attendant was given a five-digit code number so that he or she could be identified in a number of different data sets).
County
City
Birth attendant's age
Occupation as listed in census[35]
Birth attendant's own birthplace[36]
Birth attendant's parents' birthplace[37]
Year of immigration
Literacy status
Marital status
For midwives: husband's occupation[38]
Number of children listed
Age of oldest child
Age of youngest child
Household composition[39]
Number of non-family members in household
Home status (rent, mortgage, own)
Milwaukee midwife number (to link to Milwaukee Health Department data file)
State midwife number (to link to state license file)
Occupation of household head (if not husband)

This data file provided a wealth of information that contradicted many stereotypes about midwives. For example, as shown in Chapter 2, most midwives were married to artisans and had children of their own at home. In addition, many midwife families owned or mortgaged their homes, a pattern of home ownership that was consistent with those discovered by Roger Simon in his study of Milwaukee.[40] Furthermore, though the women traced to the census had been identified in other places as midwives, the census rarely listed this as their occupation. In contrast, physicians identified elsewhere were always listed in the census as physicians, an important detail that underscored the gendered meanings of professionalization in this period.

Though this data set provided unique evidence about midwives, physicians, and their families, there were several problems with using the census schedules. The chief difficulty was related to the amount of time between censuses. Because the census is taken only every ten years, many midwives and physicians who practiced in the state were missed if they took up practice and moved away in the intercensal years. This problem was particularly acute in the twenty-year period 1880–1900. Although the decade of the 1890s was a crucial decade of change for midwives, and midwives' families had the high mobility associated with artisan families, the 1890 manuscript census schedules are unavailable, as they were burned in a Washington, D.C., fire near the turn of the century. Therefore, it was not possible to link many midwives who practiced after 1880 but left the area before 1900. Furthermore, because the 1920 manuscript census was released only very recently, it was not possible to include a study of midwives and physicians who began their practice in the years after 1910. Another problem with using the census related to the "snapshot" approach. Because each midwife and physician was coded only once, changes over the life cycle of their families could not be ascertained. Though it would have been interesting to trace these families in successive censuses, the problems with locating each of them more than once precluded this kind of study.

Milwaukee City Directories

The Milwaukee city directories were used for several purposes. I generated a list of practicing midwives in Milwaukee using the section in the business directory of Wright's *Milwaukee City Directory* for the years 1870, 1875, 1881, 1885, 1890, 1895, 1900, 1905, 1911, 1915, 1919, 1925, and 1931. I noted all midwives who advertised in these years and created a list of new names for each year. I did not code these names for computer analysis, but I used them to build a list of women who practiced as midwives that I could check elsewhere.

City directories from the late nineteenth and early twentieth centuries are useful, if somewhat unreliable, sources for tracking the names of people living in cities. Most physicians listed their addresses in the city directories every year, and women who considered themselves midwives and who could afford to advertise their services were listed in the Midwives section. The listings in the years approximating census years were also useful in providing street addresses so that the midwives and the physicians could be located in the census schedules. However, the directories proved to be only of limited value, since many women who worked as midwives in Milwaukee never advertised this fact in the city directory, and many physicians listed only a named building where their office was located. These problems, combined with the known unreliability of city directories, convinced me not to use material from the Milwaukee city directories for quantitative analysis except to note the numbers of new midwives and the total number of physicians practicing in the city. Thus, no statistical tests were performed with these numbers.

The city directories were also used to trace the addresses of Milwaukee parents who had babies in the sampled months of 1900 and 1905. Because the birth certificates in these years did not provide parental addresses, an important variable in assessing the geographic location of midwives' and physicians' practices, I took the parents' names and occupations from the birth certificates and then turned to the city directories for the relevant address.

Physician Education

The birth certificate study identified a possible 1,149 physicians practicing in the four counties. To determine the medical education of these physicians, I used two sources: the state licenses filed by physicians who complied with the 1897 Medical Practice Act, and Louis Frank's Directory in his *Medical History of Milwaukee*.[41] These sources together provided details about the medical education of 912 physicians who practiced in Dane, Milwaukee, Price, and Trempealeau Counties.

Physicians' Registration and Physicians' Licenses

In 1897, a new Wisconsin statute established a Board of Medical Examiners, which was empowered to review physician qualifications to practice. Section 1435 of the Wisconsin statutes required that new practitioners register with the Board and that they present a diploma from a "reputable" medical school, defined as one that required, after 1897, a three-year program of six-month terms. An amendment in 1899 to the Practice Act required that all physicians practicing in the state register with the Board.[42] From the Physicians' Register and the Physician Licenses I was able to identify the educational credentials of 862 doctors from the four counties. Both the two-volume Register and the physician licenses that were filed after 1899 are part of the archival collection of the Board of Medical Examiners at the Archives Division of the Wisconsin State Historical Society.[43]

Unlike the midwife licenses, the physician licenses changed somewhat over time as the qualifications for practice grew increasingly strict. A 1903 amendment to the Medical Practice Act mandated that registrants be graduates of a four-year medical school, and it set preliminary requirements for prospective medical students. For the first time, doctors in Wisconsin were required to have achieved at least the requirements equal to admission to the junior year of high school before they went to medical school. After 1906, physicians were required to have had an education equal to a high school degree. A 1915 amendment (Chapter 438) raised these requirements yet again. Licensees after 1919 were required to present credentials certifying that they had had two years of college work in the basic sciences and work in either French or German. The requirements for medical school training were also stiffened. Approved medical schools were those that offered four-year courses with eight-month terms. In 1923, a new amendment (Section 147.03) mandated that applicants attest that they were acquainted with the health laws relating to communicable diseases. By 1927, Chapter 79 directed that Wisconsin physicians serve a twelve-month internship in a reputable hospital before they could receive their license.

From the register and licenses, the following variables were coded:

> Attendant number (each doctor had a unique five-digit code)
> County

City
Year of registration
Preceptor (yes or no)
Years of medical lectures (i.e., number of terms)
Medical school graduated from[44]
Year of graduation
Months in hospital (pre- or postgraduate)
Years of study (total, including preceptorship)
Years of practice (total, to date of license application)
School of practice[45]
Specialty[46]
Birthplace[47]
Earned college degree? (if noted)
Number of obstetric cases attended[48]

Frank's Medical Directory of Milwaukee

While the license and registration files provided many details about Wisconsin's physicians' education, any doctors who had ceased practice prior to 1897 did not have licenses. Louis F. Frank's "Directory of Milwaukee Physicians" provided a limited number of details for doctors who had retired from practice in Milwaukee before state licensure was mandated. From this source, I coded the following variables for fifty Milwaukee doctors:

Attendant number
County
City
Medical school graduated from
Year of graduation
School of practice
Specialty
Birthplace

Unfortunately, there was no similar source for doctors in the other three counties who ended their medical practice before 1897.

The overwhelming majority of physicians in the study, both urban and rural, were general practitioners who did not leave biographies or extensive collections of private papers. Thus, the physician data file was an invaluable source of information about a group of ordinary doctors who were practicing in an era of substantial reforms in medical education and practice. These doctors were part of the great middle of the medical profession. Most of them were neither members of the academic medical elite, nor near the bottom in terms of status and prestige. Thus, the data on physician training enabled a study of the extent of late nineteenth-century doctors' formal and apprentice training, and it provided the possibility of determining whether national educational reforms had any impact on the educational experiences of the average practitioner.

Several problems arose with these sources, however. Some of the difficulties related to how the information was noted on the physician license applications. For example, because the application asked for the number of months of hospital training in a rather ambiguous manner, some physicians wrote down only the amount of months they had spent in medical school, while others noted the months they had spent in postgraduate training in the hospital. For many doctors, the division of time between medical school and postgraduate training was unclear. Thus, I could not determine whether the hospital time the doctor noted was spent as a medical student or as an intern, or if the time was a total of both medical school and postgraduate training. Therefore, the amounts noted on the license applications were coded as the number of months of hospital time spent either pre- or postgraduate.

Other problems related to the way in which the form changed over time. Because of this, it was not possible to obtain complete information on every variable for every physician. The best example of this problem is the variable that coded for the number of obstetrical cases attended. Prior to 1912, the license application did not ask for information about obstetrical training, so there is no such information for physicians who received their licenses prior to this date. Beginning in 1912, the form included a line that asked for the number of obstetric cases attended "under proper supervision." However, the license applications were not consistent in requiring registrants to note the number of obstetrical cases that they had overseen, nor were registrants consistent in reporting the number of cases they had attended even when the licenses asked for the information. This problem may have related to the fact that this line was never mandated by any of the Wisconsin statutes relating to medical practice. Instead, Dr. John Beffel, who served on the Board of Medical Examiners during the second decade of the twentieth century, took credit for instituting a policy that followed the recommendations of a prominent Philadelphia obstetrician and educator.[49] Between 1912 and 1917, the license forms asked for the number of obstetrical cases overseen, yet 34 of the 101 registrants in these years did not report this information. Between 1918 and 1930, the forms only sporadically asked for this information, and thus only 20 of 47 licenses reported the number of obstetrical cases overseen. Another problem related to the question of premedical education. Though amendments to the Medical Practice Act after 1904 added increasingly strict requirements concerning premedical education, these data were reported only sporadically on the license applications. Therefore, though the earning of an undergraduate degree was coded, any analysis of premedical education would have been incomplete and perhaps unrepresentative.

Frank's medical directory was certainly helpful in tracing Milwaukee doctors who stopped practicing before 1897. However, the amount of information from that source was limited to the medical school and the graduation date. In addition, the directory must be used with caution, as some of the details may be inaccurate. When I compared information from the physician license applications to that from Frank's directory, I found some details from the latter source to be incorrect.

Data Analysis

All of the information sources were hand-coded and then made ready for machine processing. To analyze the data, I used various subroutines of SPSS-PC, a popular and reliable statistical package. For the underlying statistical assumptions regarding a particular statistical analysis, I refer the reader to the various handbooks supporting this program.[50]

Though most of the data sets presented no particular problems, when the birth data set was aggregated by attendant number, a problem arose that related to its distribution and indirectly to some of the assumptions underlying statistical analysis. Because most midwives and doctors delivered very few births, the data assumed a

Poisson distribution. This nonnormal probability distribution is typical of probability functions using discrete integers that describe such phenomena as demand for services (for example, the services of birth attendants). In many cases, the fact that the Poisson distribution is nonnormal would require that the data be analyzed by procedures not relying on normal distributions. However, when the number (n) is large and the probability (p) is small, the Poisson distribution approximates the binomial distribution, and most familiar tests of significance may be used.[51]

Notes

❧

Introduction

1. For the drop in midwife-attended births, see Judith Walzer Leavitt, *Brought to Bed: Childbearing in America, 1750–1950* (New York: Oxford University Press, 1986), p. 12, graph. According to Judy Barrett Litoff, by 1930 at least 80 percent of all midwives were reported to be living in the south. Judy Barrett Litoff, *American Midwives, 1860 to the Present,* Contributions in Medical History, no. 1 (Westport, Conn.: Greenwood Press, 1978), p. 141.

2. Nurse-midwives, registered nurses who receive further training for attending childbirth, encountered many negative stereotypes when they began to try to attract middle-class patients in the 1950s and 1960s. Wrote one nurse-midwife, midwifery "conjured up images of old women with dirty hands and stained clothes, delivering babies in hovels while burning herbs at the foot of the bed." Barbara Brennan and Joan Rattner Hellman, *The Complete Book of Midwifery* (New York: Dutton, 1973), p. 12; quoted in Margot Edwards and Mary Waldorf, *Reclaiming Birth: History and Heroines of American Childbirth Reform* (Trumansburg, N.Y.: The Crossing Press, 1984), p. 155.

3. In addition to Leavitt, *Brought to Bed,* see Richard W. Wertz and Dorothy C. Wertz, *Lying-In: A History of Childbirth in America* (New York: Free Press, 1977); Catherine M. Scholten, *Childbearing in American Society, 1650–1850* (New York: New York University Press, 1985); and Sylvia D. Hoffert, *Private Matters: American Attitudes toward Childbearing and Infant Nurture in the Urban North, 1800–1860* (Urbana: University of Illinois Press, 1989).

4. One of the most influential books on the Progressive Era in general is Robert H. Wiebe, *The Search for Order, 1877–1920* (New York: Hill and Wang, 1967). Paul Starr's work has become the standard for its excellent discussion of science and medicine in this period. See Starr, *The Social Transformation of American Medicine: The Rise of a Sovereign Profession and the Making of a Vast Industry* (New York: Basic Books, 1982), esp. pp. 140–144. Irvine Loudon's recent study of maternal mortality examines the statistics that were used to evaluate risk. He finds little movement in the overall maternal mortality rate until the late 1930s, well after physicians had replaced midwives in many countries. See Loudon, *Death in Childbirth: An International Study of Maternal Care and Maternal Mortality 1800–1950* (New York: Clarendon Press, Oxford, 1992).

5. One of the most famous obstetricians of this period, Joseph B. DeLee, described the struggle between midwives and physicians in terms of elevating science. Midwives, he argued, were "relics of barbarism." DeLee, "Progress toward Ideal Obstetrics," *American Journal of Obstetrics and Diseases of Women and Children* 73 (1916): 407–415.

6. Magali Sarfatti Larson discusses these criteria in her *Rise of Professionalism: A Sociological Analysis* (Berkeley: University of California Press, 1977), pp. 17, 41–45.

7. Eliot Freidson, "Are Professions Necessary?" in Thomas Haskell, ed., *The Authority of Experts: Studies in History and Theory* (Bloomington: Indiana University Press, 1984), p. 10.

8. Haskell, *The Authority of Experts,* "Introduction," pp. x–xviii, 5. Burton J. Bledstein, in *The Culture of Professionalism* (New York: Norton, 1976), argues that professionalization became a strategy used by individuals who wished to protect themselves against the rigid employment patterns of nineteenth-century capitalism.

9. Leavitt *(Brought to Bed),* Hoffert *(Private Matters),* and Sally G. McMillen *(Motherhood in the Old South: Pregnancy, Childbirth, and Infant Rearing,* Baton Rouge: Louisiana State University Press, 1990) all show that white, middle-class, native-born women hired physicians for their confinements as early as the beginning of the nineteenth century.

10. Elizabeth Ewen, *Immigrant Women in the Land of Dollars: Life and Culture on the Lower East Side* (New York: Monthly Review Press, 1985), explores these roles for immigrant women in New York City. See especially Chapter 8, "In Sickness and in Health," pp. 130–146. As the text of succeeding chapters reveals, I found very few physicians to be female. Furthermore, as several authors have noted, this period was one in which the number of women physicians declined significantly. See, for example, Regina Markell Morantz-Sanchez, *Sympathy and Science: Women Physicians in American Medicine* (New York: Oxford University Press, 1985), pp. 232–265, and Mary Roth Walsh, *"Doctors Wanted: No Women Need Apply": Sexual Barriers in the Medical Profession, 1835–1975* (New Haven: Yale University Press, 1977), pp. 159–165.

11. See George Rosen (Charles E. Rosenberg, ed.), *The Structure of American Medical Practice, 1875–1941* (Philadelphia: University of Pennsylvania Press, 1983).

12. See, for example, Larson, *The Rise of Professionalism;* Eliot Freidson, *Profession of Medicine* (New York: Harper and Row, 1970); and Starr, *Social Transformation of American Medicine.*

13. See Barbara Melosh, *"The Physician's Hand": Work Culture and Conflict in American Nursing* (Philadelphia: Temple University Press, 1982).

14. Susan M. Reverby examines the effect of gender on attempts to professionalize nursing; see Reverby, *Ordered to Care: The Dilemma of American Nursing, 1850–1945* (New York: Cambridge University Press, 1987). Barbara Melosh examines the interaction of gender and work in nursing's professional process; see *"The Physician's Hand".* Nancy Tomes found that nursing school superintendents saw one of their principal duties as turning out middle-class young women; see her " 'Little World of Our Own': The Pennsylvania Hospital Training School for Nurses, 1895–1907," *Journal of the History of Medicine and Allied Sciences* 33 (1978): 507–530.

15. Historians and sociologists have differed on the relationship between power and professionalism. Eliot Freidson argues that experts, who have special skills and knowledge, also acquire power and prestige. See Friedson, "Are the Professions Nec-

essary?" in Haskell, *The Authority of Experts,* pp. 3–25. Magali Larson, in *The Rise of Professionalism,* sees the class issue as preceding the professional one. Antonio Gramsci is widely quoted for his work on cultural hegemony, the ability by professionals and others to exert power in the absence of coercion; see Joseph Femia, "Hegemony and Consciousness in the Thought of Antonio Gramsci," *Political Studies* 23, 1 (1975): 29–48. JoAnne Brown reminds us of the power of language in claiming professional power; see her "Professional Language: Words that Succeed," *Radical History Review* 34 (1986): 33–51. Darlene Clark Hine's analysis of black nurses is one the few attempts to examine the interaction of gender and race or ethnicity. Nursing, she argues, was one of the more accessible of the professions for black women, and it enabled a black woman from the working class to rise into the middle class. She points out, however, that black nurses were rigidly segregated, and expected only to serve the black community. But the black community gave these women an enormous amount of respect. See Hine's *Black Women in White: Racial Conflict and Cooperation in the Nursing Profession, 1890–1950* (Bloomington: Indiana University Press, 1989].

16. "Catching" babies is a slang term with old and somewhat nebulous roots. The term probably is traceable historically to neighbor-woman midwives, and its meaning suggests a birth attendant who sat by and did not interfere with the birth. Even today, lay midwives and even some doctors will use the term to discuss how many babies they have delivered. The *Dictionary of American Regional English* notes that the word "catch" has been used in the south and southeast by both midwives and doctors to denote the assisting of the delivery of a baby. Interestingly, the word also has been used in many places in the United States to mean "to become pregnant." Frederic G. Cassidy, ed. *Dictionary of American Regional English* (Cambridge: Belknap Press of Harvard University Press, 1985), vol. 1, p. 561.

17. For an excellent discussion of the evolution of this concept of safety, see Leavitt, *Brought to Bed,* pp. 36–63.

18. See Starr, *Social Transformation of American Medicine;* Kenneth M. Ludmerer, *Learning to Heal: The Development of American Medical Education* (New York: Basic Books, 1985); William G. Rothstein, *American Medical Schools and the Practice of Medicine: A History* (New York: Oxford University Press, 1987); Ronald L. Numbers, ed., *The Education of American Physicians: Historical Essays* (Berkeley: University of California Press, 1980); and Martin Kaufman, *American Medical Education: The Formative Years, 1765–1910* (Westport, Conn.: Greenwood Press, 1976).

19. Edward Atwater examined a group of physicians who practiced in Rochester, New York, in the nineteenth century. His work mentioned the training of doctors who practiced in the city, but he was more interested in their professional alliances and the rise of medical institutions in Rochester. See Edward C. Atwater, "The Medical Profession in a New Society, Rochester, New York (1811–60)," *Bulletin of the History of Medicine* 47 (1973): 221–235; and "The Physicians of Rochester, N.Y., 1860–1910: A Study in Professional History, II," *Bulletin of the History of Medicine* 47 (1973): 93–106.

20. Judith Walzer Leavitt discusses this gap between the reality of obstetric training and the perceptions of scientific competence. However, Leavitt's interest lies more with women's perceptions, and she does not systematically investigate physician training. See Leavitt, *Brought to Bed.*

21. Though there was no separate blank on the state midwife license applications

to indicate the number of cases attended while in school, many applicants made a point to note this fact, particularly those women who attended midwife schools in Milwaukee. The number of cases varied widely, ranging from a midwife who attended twelve cases in school to a 1913 graduate who oversaw forty-one (Board of Medical Examiners, Midwife File, Series 1611, Archives Division, Wisconsin State Historical Society, Madison, Wisconsin).

22. Though physicians rationalized their assumption of these cases in terms of objective, professional science, this process really embodied an older ideal of therapeutic efficacy based on a shared world view between the doctor and the patient. See Charles E. Rosenberg, "The Therapeutic Revolution: Medicine, Meaning, and Social Change in Nineteenth-Century America," in Morris J. Vogel and Charles E. Rosenberg, eds., *The Therapeutic Revolution: Essays in the Social History of American Medicine* (Philadelphia: University of Pennsylvania Press, 1979), pp. 3–26; and John Harley Warner, *The Therapeutic Perspective: Medical Practice, Knowledge, and Identity in America, 1820–1885* (Cambridge: Harvard University Press, 1986).

23. Morantz-Sanchez points out that women doctors in this period were shut out of the growing "scientific" specialties. In response, they argued that this laboratory model increased the emotional distance between doctors and patients, threatening the humanity of the physician. But the laboratory model, championed by such prominent educators as William Welch at Johns Hopkins, represented "scientific medicine," and it helped to improve the overall standing of medicine in the twentieth century. This new model of practice denied the necessity of the humane qualities women doctors had brought to the profession, and left little place for them. See Morantz-Sanchez, *Sympathy and Science,* pp. 238–241.

24. I used data from four counties that ranged from urban to rural to frontier. Milwaukee was a representative urban, industrial city, and its political, social, and even public health history have been well documented. Dane County was a settled rural area, the site of Madison, the state's capitol city. Trempealeau County, the subject of Merle Curti's famous analysis of frontier democracy, was a settled rural county with many European immigrant farmers. See Curti, *The Making of an American Community: A Case Study of Democracy in a Frontier County,* with the assistance of Robert Daniel et al. (Stanford: Stanford University Press, 1959). Price County in northern Wisconsin, settled only in the last decades of the nineteenth century, was a frontier area, one of the state's early logging counties and a site of the midwest timber industry.

25. Massachusetts banned midwifery in one section of the Medical Practice Act of 1894. As Eugene Declerq and Richard Lacroix have shown, midwives continued to practice in Lawrence, Massachusetts, until about 1914. However, when the state began to prosecute them, midwives stopped filing birth certificates under their own names, so it is difficult to know if the decline in midwife-attended births was real or an artifact of the data collection procedures. See Declerq and Lacroix, "The Immigrant Midwives of Lawrence: The Conflict between Law and Culture in Early Twentieth-Century Massachusetts," *Bulletin of the History of Medicine* 59 (1985): 232–246. Many southern states, on the other hand, did not begin to regulate midwifery practice until after World War I. This lack of regulation undoubtedly was due to racism, as most southern midwives were African-American. However, while leaving midwives free to practice, these states also had no way of counting the number of

births in each state. See Onnie Lee Logan as told to Katherine Clark, *Motherwit: An Alabama Midwife's Story* (New York: E. P. Dutton, 1989).

26. For an analysis of some of the specifics in the history of medicine in the state, see the group of essays in Ronald L. Numbers and Judith Walzer Leavitt, eds., *Wisconsin Medicine: Historical Perspectives* (Madison: University of Wisconsin Press, 1981).

27. See, for example, Frances E. Kobrin, "The American Midwife Controversy: A Crisis of Professionalization," *Bulletin of the History of Medicine* 40 (1966): 350–363; reprinted in Judith Walzer Leavitt, ed., *Women and Health in America: Historical Readings* (Madison: University of Wisconsin Press, 1984), pp. 318–326. See also Judy Barrett Litoff, *American Midwives;* and Jane B. Donegan, " 'Safe Delivered,' But by Whom? Midwives and Men-Midwives in Early America," in Leavitt, *Women and Health in America,* pp. 302–317. Laurel Thatcher Ulrich, in her article " 'The Living Mother of a Living Child': Midwifery and Mortality in Post-Revolutionary New England," *William and Mary Quarterly,* 3rd Series, 46 (1989): 27–48, and her prizewinning book, *A Midwife's Tale: The Life of Martha Ballard, Based on Her Diary, 1785–1812* (New York: Alfred A. Knopf, 1990) examined the Ballard diary and other evidence, and found that in 1800, Mrs. Ballard was the most important practitioner in her town. For studies of later periods, see Neal Devitt, "The Statistical Case for Elimination of the Midwife: Fact versus Prejudice, 1890–1935," *Women and Health* 4 (1979): 81–96; 169–186; Declerq and Lacroix, "The Immigrant Midwives of Lawrence"; and Eugene Declerq, "The Nature and Style of Practice of Immigrant Midwives in Early Twentieth-Century Massachusetts," *Journal of Social History* 19 (1985): 113–129.

28. Eugene Declerq points out the paucity of work that focuses on the actual practice of midwifery. See Declerq, "The Nature and Style of Practice," p. 113.

29. Judy Litoff emphasizes the cultural and language differences among midwives that helped to keep them from forming groups on their own behalf. Midwives, she argues, were reliant upon others to organize them or to write articles about midwife affairs. At the same time, physician opponents to midwives were better organized and more articulate. See Litoff, *American Midwives,* pp. 106–107, 113.

30. Eugene Declerq's work on Lawrence, Massachusetts, concentrates on immigrant midwives. He analyzes the practice of "active" midwives in the city and finds that most midwives based their practice in their immediate neighborhoods. Declerq does not examine the practice of physicians who lived in these neighborhoods, however (Declerq, "The Nature and Style of Practice").

31. See, for example, Barbara Ehrenreich and Deidre English, *Witches, Midwives, and Nurses: A History of Women Healers* (Oyster Bay, N.Y.: Glass Mountain Pamphlets, 1973); and G. J. Barker-Benfield, *The Horrors of the Half-Known Life: Male Attitudes toward Women and Sexuality in Nineteenth-Century America* (New York: Harper and Row, 1976).

32. Jane Pacht Brickman, "Public Health, Midwives, and Nurses, 1880–1930," in Ellen Condliffe Lagemann, ed., *Nursing History: New Perspectives, New Possibilities* (New York: Teacher's College Press, 1983), pp. 65–88.

33. Leavitt, *Brought to Bed.*

34. Ulrich, *A Midwife's Tale,* p. 33.

35. For a good summary of these issues, see Clyde Griffen, "Review Essay: Com-

181

munity Studies and the Investigation of Nineteenth-Century Social Relations," *Social Science History* 10 (1986): 315–316.

36. Kathleen Neils Conzen, *Immigrant Milwaukee, 1836–1860: Accommodation and Community in a Frontier City,* Harvard Studies in Urban History (Cambridge: Harvard University Press, 1976); Olivier Zunz, *The Changing Face of Inequality: Urbanization, Industrial Development, and Immigrants in Detroit, 1880–1920* (Chicago: University of Chicago Press, 1982. See also John Bodnar, Roger Simon, and Michael P. Weber, *Lives of Their Own: Blacks, Italians, and Poles in Pittsburgh, 1900–1960* (Urbana: University of Illinois Press, 1982) and John J. Bukowczyk, "Polish Rural Culture and Immigrant Working Class Formation, 1880–1914," *Polish American Studies* 41 (1984): 23–44. Unlike the other works mentioned above, Kathleen Conzen's study of Milwaukee focuses on the mid-nineteenth century, but her conclusions about the dynamic nature of ethnic neighborhoods is the same.

37. Zunz, *The Changing Face of Inequality,* p. 4.

38. Robert H. Wiebe, in *The Search for Order,* describes professionals as an important constituent of the new middle class of the late nineteenth century (pp. 111–132). See also Starr, *Social Transformation of American Medicine.*

39. Richard Hofstadter's important analysis of the Progressive period used this approach. He argued that the foreign-born took a dim view of Progressive reformers. These reformers, in the eyes of the immigrant community, stood for bizarre or even offensive ideas like women's rights, temperance, and Sunday blue laws. Hofstadter maintains that the abstractions of the Progressives, such as efficiency, good government, and businesslike management, had no appeal within the immigrant experience. See Richard Hofstadter, *The Age of Reform: From Bryan to F. D. R.* (New York: Random House, 1955)]. Robert Wiebe, in *The Search for Order,* argued that Progressives came from a "new middle class" of far-sighted physicians, businessmen, scientists, engineers, and social workers who were determined to use their knowledge and skills to solve the problems caused by industrialization and to impose order on a chaotic society. Though some early studies had found nativist tendencies among the Progressives, John Higham's influential study of immigrants argues that the Progressives were tolerant towards immigrant groups. Indeed, Progressive reformers were optimistic about immigrants' contributions to American society, though Higham admits that the contributions that were admired were usually small and inconsequential. See Higham, *Strangers in the Land: Patterns of American Nativism, 1860–1925* (New Brunswick: Rutgers University Press, 1955)]. Some recent work has criticized Hofstadter, Wiebe, and Higham for their emphasis on the elite leaders of the Progressive movement and for failing to define just who were the "middle class." They have also been criticized for underestimating the contributions of farmers, workers, and immigrants. See the discussion in Arthur S. Link and Richard L. McCormick, *Progressivism* (Arlington Heights, Ill.: Harlan Davidson, 1983), pp. 7–9.

1. Training Midwives

1. License application of Bertha Wichtel, Board of Medical Examiners, Midwife File, Series 1611, Archives Division, Wisconsin State Historical Society, Madison, Wisconsin (hereafter referred to as Midwife File, WSHS).

2. License application of Dora Larson, Midwife File, WSHS.

3. The literature on the reform of medical and nursing education is substantial. For educational reform in nursing, see Susan M. Reverby, *Ordered to Care: The Dilemma of American Nursing, 1850–1945* (New York: Cambridge University Press, 1987); and Barbara Melosh, *"The Physician's Hand": Work Culture and Conflict in American Nursing* (Philadelphia: Temple University Press, 1987). For educational reform and professional status in medicine, see Paul Starr, *The Social Transformation of American Medicine: The Rise of a Sovereign Profession and the Making of a Vast Industry* (New York: Basic Books, 1982); Kenneth M. Ludmerer, *Learning to Heal: The Development of American Medical Education* (New York: Basic Books, 1985); William G. Rothstein, *American Medical Schools and the Practice of Medicine: A History* (New York: Oxford University Press, 1987); and Charles E. Rosenberg, *The Care of Strangers: The Rise of America's Hospital System* (New York: Basic Books, 1987).

4. Frances E. Kobrin was the first to suggest that midwifery faced a crisis of professionalization. However, Kobrin found this crisis within medicine, not within midwifery. See Kobrin, "The American Midwife Controversy: A Crisis of Professionalization," *Bulletin of the History of Medicine* 40 (1966): 350–363.

5. These midwives were often referred to as "granny" midwives. However, the word "granny" is both an unspecific and politically loaded term. It often referred to any old woman practicing midwifery, regardless of her training. More important, "granny" carries a politically charged meaning with ageist overtones. In their attempts to discredit the knowledge midwives gained through long experience, turn-of-the-century critics of midwifery often contemptuously referred to any woman practicing midwifery as a "granny." Even today, the term is still problematic, and I have avoided its use in this study.

6. License application of Susan Washburn, Midwife File, WSHS.

7. The training and midwifery experience of Susan Washburn and other neighbor women was very much like that of Martha Ballard, a Maine midwife who practiced at the end of the eighteenth century. See Laurel Thatcher Ulrich in *A Midwife's Tale: The Life of Martha Ballard, Based on Her Diary, 1785–1812* (New York: Alfred A. Knopf, 1990).

8. Molly Ladd-Taylor, " 'Grannies' and 'Spinsters': Midwife Education under the Sheppard-Towner Act," *Journal of Social History* 22 (Winter 1988): 261.

9. Elizabeth G. Fox, "Rural Problems," in Children's Bureau, *Standards of Child Welfare: A Report of the Children's Bureau Conferences, May and June 1919*, U.S. Department of Labor, Children's Bureau Publication no. 60 (Washington, D.C.: Government Printing Office, 1919), p. 187.

10. Ladd-Taylor, " 'Grannies' and 'Spinsters,' " p. 263.

11. A one-way analysis of variance (ANOVA) of age by kind of training was highly significant. The F-value equaled 7.7251, with a significance of 0.00001.

12. James Lincoln Huntington, "The Midwives of Massachusetts," *Boston Medical and Surgical Journal* 167 (1912): 542–548. Huntington's data are quite crude. The information was collected by various social work agencies throughout Massachusetts, and the tables in his article present the data in summary form. To analyze the ages of midwives lacking diplomas, only those columns where age and training could be linked were used. Among the four usable tables, 24 midwives were identified by age and lack of diplomas.

13. All of the licenses (373) were examined and coded for computer analysis. Using the popular program SPSS (Statistical Package for the Social Sciences) to analyze the

data, *t*-tests to evaluate differences in mean age were run between the different groups. The *t*-test comparing the mean age of those reporting school training and those reporting no school training was highly significant, with a *t* value of −4.56 and a significance level (2-tail) of .00001. To investigate the link between region and type of midwife, the 52 counties represented by the registrants were grouped into six regions. When these six regions were cross-tabulated with kind of training, the result was highly significant: $X^2 = -102.33$, with 15 degrees of freedom (df), and a significance level of .00001. Particular individual cells contributed to this finding: the western and central regions had three times more than the expected number of midwives reporting "no training," and the city of Milwaukee, where twenty midwives reporting "no training" would be expected, in fact had only one.

14. Physicians' Register, City of Milwaukee Health Department, Archives Section, Milwaukee Public Library (hereafter Milwaukee Health Department, Physicians' Register). The title of this registry is a misnomer, for it contains registration data on both physicians and midwives. Between June 1877 and October 1907, 658 entries for midwives were made, but many of the women who registered in 1906 and 1907 had entered their names previously. All told, the Register provided information on 588 different women. There were no discernable trends in when these women registered. One or two neighbor-woman midwives in Milwaukee signed up with the Health Department every year. The figures were as follows:

	1877–1879	1880–1889	1890–1899	1900–1907
Total registered	46	171	227	144
"No training"	6	0	3	12

15. A Children's Bureau study of Marathon County, Wisconsin, described a German midwife, Mrs. R., practicing there who had trained herself by reading a text on midwifery that she had brought with her from Germany. As the mother of eleven children, she relied a great deal on her own experience. As described by the authors, Mrs. R. was a typical neighbor-woman midwife: five of the sixteen births she attended were those of her own grandchildren, although she did oversee a few cases for her neighbors, for which she was paid. Florence Brown Sherbon and Elizabeth Moore, *Maternity and Infant Care in Two Rural Counties in Wisconsin,* U.S. Department of Labor, Children's Bureau Publication no. 46 (Washington, D.C.: Government Printing Office, 1919), p. 34.

16. In Marathon County, Wisconsin, for example, many areas were served by minor roads, which were impassable to autos and difficult even for wagons. In addition, many parts of the county had no mail delivery; some people had to travel twelve miles for their mail. Sherbon and Moore, *Maternity and Infant Care,* pp. 20–22.

17. License application of Mrs. Minnie Gray, Midwife File, WSHS.

18. License application of Anne Nowak, Midwife File, WSHS.

19. Onnie Lee Logan as told to Katherine Clark, *Motherwit: An Alabama Midwife's Story* (New York: E. P. Dutton, 1989), pp. 88, 84.

20. Onnie Lee Logan's grandmother, for example, was a slave midwife, and her mother also practiced midwifery. Logan, *Motherwit,* pp. 47–50. See also Linda Janet Holmes, "Louvenia Taylor Benjamin, Southern Lay Midwife: An Interview," *Sage* 2, no. 2 (Fall 1985): 52; also Debra Anne Susie, *In the Way of Our Grandmothers: A*

Cultural View of Twentieth-Century Midwifery in Florida (Athens: University of Georgia Press, 1988), pp. 18–19.

21. License application of Mary Greeley, Midwife File, WSHS.

22. License application of Ellen Stiefvator, Midwife File, WSHS.

23. License application of Gabrielle Sedall, Midwife File, WSHS.

24. License application of Ellen Stiefvator, Midwife File, WSHS.

25. License applications of Mary A. Weidman of Marshfield and Mary Gordan of Arkensaw, Midwife File, WSHS.

26. Holmes, "Louvenia Taylor Benjamin," p. 52.

27. Quoted in Sherbon and Moore, *Maternity and Infant Care,* p. 33.

28. Jane Pacht Brickman's study of the campaign against midwives in the early twentieth century asserts that "medical animus against the midwife focused on the urban practitioner." See Brickman, "Public Health, Midwives, and Nurses, 1880–1930," in Ellen Condliffe Lagemann, ed., *Nursing History: New Perspectives, New Possibilities* (New York: Teacher's College Press, 1983), p. 70.

29. License applications for both the city of Milwaukee and the state of Wisconsin required two physician references. Each woman's references were coded, and names of physicians in selected counties were checked against their own license applications (Board of Medical Examiners, Physician Licenses, Series 1606, Archives Division, Wisconsin State Historical Society, Madison, Wisconsin; hereafter known as Physician Licenses, WSHS). For physicians' activities within the medical community, I consulted Louis F. Frank, *The Medical History of Milwaukee, 1834–1914* (Milwaukee: Germania Publishing Co., 1915).

30. License application of Frances Jahnz, Midwife File, WSHS. See Chapter 7 for an extended discussion of Dr. Wasielewski's own obstetrical practice in Milwaukee's Polish community.

31. License application of Mary Browikowski, Midwife File, WSHS.

32. License application of Henriette Wenzel, Midwife File, WSHS. Hinz practiced in Milwaukee from 1875 to 1903. Frank, *Medical History of Milwaukee,* p. 255.

33. State license applicants reported four other Milwaukee physicians who offered lectures. Some of these doctors later were instrumental in the founding of several midwifery schools in Milwaukee. See license applications of Kondaneygli Sythowski, Helena F. Mueller, Frericka Wirth, and Mary Dudek, Midwife File, WSHS.

34. License application of Mary Holub, Midwife File, WSHS.

35. Magali Sarfatti Larson, *The Rise of Professionalism: A Sociological Analysis* (Berkeley: University of California Press, 1977), pp.44–45.

36. Ibid., p. 45.

37. Ibid., p. 17.

38. Ibid., p. 41. Larson cites the studies of Haroun Jamous and B. Peloille, "Changes in the French University-Hospital System," in J. A. Jackson, ed., *Professions and Professionalization,* (Cambridge: Cambridge University Press, 1970), pp. 111–112.

39. Paul Starr, *The Social Transformation of American Medicine,* pp. 109–120.

40. See the extended discussion in Reverby, *Ordered to Care.*

41. Janet Wilson James, "Isabel Hampton and Professionalization of Nursing in the 1890s," in Morris J. Vogel and Charles E. Rosenberg, eds., *The Therapeutic Revolution: Essays in the Social History of Medicine* (Philadelphia: University of Pennsylvania Press, 1979), pp. 201–244.

42. Melosh, *"The Physician's Hand,"* p. 38.

43. Ibid., p. 4.

44. Erna Lesky, *The Vienna Medical School of the Nineteenth Century,* trans. L. Williams and I. S. Levij (Baltimore: Johns Hopkins University Press, 1976), p. 190.

45. H. MacNaughton-Jones, "The Royal School for Midwives at Munich," *The Hospital,* June 28, 1902, 227–229. also Arthur B. Emmons and James L. Huntington, "Has the Trained and Supervised Midwife Made Good?" *Transactions for the American Association for the Study and the Prevention of Infant Mortality* 2 (1911): 202.

46. Agnes C. Vietor, ed., *A Woman's Quest: The Life of Marie E. Zakrzewska, M.D.* (New York: D. Appleton, 1924), p. 38.

47. S. Josephine Baker, "Schools for Midwives," *Transactions of the American Association for the Study and the Prevention of Infant Mortality* 2 (1911): 232–248. German schools are discussed on pp. 234–237, French on p. 237. A massive Children's Bureau study of European childbirth customs included surveys of midwifery training. See Nettie McGill, *Infant-Welfare Work in Europe: An Account of Recent Experiences in Great Britain [sic], Austria, Belgium, France, Germany, and Italy,* U.S. Department of Labor, Children's Bureau Publication no. 76 (Washington, D.C.: Government Printing Office, 1921), "France," p. 83. Some scholarships were available to needy students; for example, in France, a municipal government might occasionally sponsor a student.

48. McGill, *Infant-Welfare Work in Europe.* See also Baker, "Schools for Midwives," pp. 234–237. The course at Vienna in the middle of the nineteenth century lasted five months (Lesky, *Vienna Medical School,* p. 423).

49. An 1818 German statute allowed only educated midwives to practice and required that midwives call a physician in any case of abnormal labor (Vietor, *A Woman's Quest,* pp. 37–38). French midwives were also required to have either a first- or a second-class license. The latter required less schooling, but a holder of a second-class license could practice only in the department where she trained. McGill, "France," *Infant-Welfare Work in Europe).* Denmark, Sweden, and Norway required practicing midwives to take refresher courses. See George W. Kosmak, "Results of Supervised Midwife Practice in Certain European Countries," *Journal of the American Medical Association* 89 (1927): 2009–2010.

50. By 1910, Polish immigrants constituted at least one-fifth of the total foreign-born population of Milwaukee. The 1910 census did not break down the foreign-born population by country of origin and year of arrival, but it is likely that most of the Polish foreign-born population had lived in the city ten years or less Roger Simon, "The Expansion of an Industrial City: Milwaukee, 1880–1910" (Ph.D. diss., University of Wisconsin—Madison, 1971), p. 82.

51. Agnes Pradzinska, letter to the editor, *American Midwife* (St. Louis), German language edition, 2, 6 (1896): 40–41. My thanks to Rebecca Bohling for her expert help in translating this letter for me.

52. Dr. John Winters Brannan, "Report of the Bellevue Midwife School, from August 1, 1911, to August 1, 1915," cited in J. Clifton Edgar, "The Education, Licensing and Supervision of the Midwife," *American Journal of Obstetrics and Diseases of Women and Children* 73 (1916): 392.

53. The labor for a woman having her first baby is usually longer than the labor for a multiparous woman. Thus, a primipara historically was considered at higher risk during labor and delivery.

54. J. Clifton Edgar, "Why the Midwife?" *American Journal of Obstetrics* 78 (1918): 247. Judy Barrett Litoff describes other well-regarded curricula at the Playfair School in Chicago and the College of Midwifery at St. Louis. See Litoff, *American Midwives, 1860 to the Present,* Contributions in Medical History, no. 1 (Westport, Conn.: Greenwood Press, 1978), pp. 35–37.

55. Grace Abbott, *The Immigrant and the Community* (New York: Century Co., 1917), p. 152.

56. Though literacy was not a necessary qualification for practice, most of Wisconsin's midwives, like other northern midwives, were literate in some language. In the census study, of the 359 cases where literacy could be ascertained, 343 midwives (95.5 percent) were described as able to read or write. Only 16 women in this sample were not literate. Eugene Declerq's study of Lawrence, Massachusetts, midwives also found a high degree of literacy among midwives. He cites a 1909 study by the Research Department of the Boston School for Social Workers that found that 80 percent of Lawrence midwives were literate. See Declerq, "The Nature and Style of Practice of Immigrant Midwives in Early Twentieth Century Massachusetts," *Journal of Social History* 19 (1985): 118.

57. The St. Louis School of Midwives offered classes in English and German from 1874 to 1877, but then dropped the English classes due to a lack of demand. The school attracted large numbers of German immigrant women in St. Louis who were attracted to the school. See Diana S. Perry, "The Early Midwives of Missouri," *Journal of Nurse-Midwifery* 28 (November–December 1983): 16.

58. Advertisement, *American Midwife* (St. Louis) 1, 1 (1896): 6. The Bellevue School, serving one of the most polyglot populations in the United States, taught its course primarily in English, although its founders did initially attempt to find doctors and nurses who spoke German and Italian and could instruct midwife pupils in their own language. See John Winters Brannan, "Opportunities for the Education of Midwives," *American Journal of Obstetrics* 63 (1911): 900–901.

59. Simon, "Expansion of an Industrial City," p. 60, Table 3–1.

60. Simon, "Expansion of an Industrial City," pp. 82, 83.

61. The State License file also showed the wide influence on Wisconsin's midwives: of the 121 women in the state file who reported that their school was based in Milwaukee, 30 gave addresses outside of the city. Bertha Schmidt of Appleton, Wisconsin, for example, stated, "For 10 years before going to school I attended confinement cases with doctors in my county. Then went to school and completed the course in three months of classwork." She graduated from the Milwaukee School of Midwifery in 1896 (Midwife File, WSHS).

62. As is the case with many proprietary schools of the era, there are no surviving records from the midwifery schools in Milwaukee. Piecing together disparate sources, I found information about Wilhelmine Stein's education through her own registration with the Milwaukee Health Department in 1879. For Stein's personal history, I found useful data in the manuscript censuses of 1880 and 1900.

63. Frank, "Charles W. Betzel," *Medical History of Milwaukee,* p. 247. Betzel practiced medicine in Milwaukee until he retired in 1888. He died there in 1895.

64. Alphonse Kalckhoff, Physician Licenses, WSHS.

65. Wright's *Milwaukee City Directory* (Milwaukee: Alfred G. Wright, 1891–1894). Listed under "Lying-In Institutes."

66. License application of Rosalia Noll, Midwife File, WSHS.

67. License application of Anna Schreiber, Midwife File, WSHS.

68. License application of Caroline Kueny, Midwife File, WSHS.

69. See Reverby, *Ordered to Care,* esp. Chapter 4, –pp. 60–76.

70. License application of Sophia Kegel, Midwife File, WSHS.

71. Marie Walentauska, a 1902 graduate of the Milwaukee School of Midwifery, reported having this coursework. Josephine Fries, a 1904 graduate, reported having a nine-month course with nine months of "hospital work at the same school." Midwife File, WSHS.

72. Sophia Kegel, Midwife File, WSHS.

73. An article in the *Milwaukee Sentinel* reporting on one of the school's graduations noted that Drs. Kalckchoff and Betzell had awarded diplomas to several "Mesdames" and one "Miss." "Diplomas Awarded by Milwaukee Institute for Midwifery," *Milwaukee Sentinel,* January 6, 1886, p. 2.

74. Milwaukee Health Department, Physicians' Register, 1883. Schenermann had graduated from the medical school at Wurzburg in 1855. See entry for August 31, 1882, Milwaukee Health Department, Physicians' Register.

75. Dr. Alois Graettinger, who had been privately instructing midwives in Milwaukee for several years, trained in medicine at the Faculty University at Munich, Germany, in 1878. Registering with the Milwaukee Health Department in 1882, his office was in the same neighborhood as another founder, Dr. William Schorse. Schorse, also a recent émigré to Wisconsin, had received his medical degree from the University of Goettingen in 1877. Dr. William Meyer, the third physician, was the only one of the three with an American medical degree. He had graduated from Rush Medical College in 1879 (Milwaukee Health Department, Physicians' Register). Graettinger went on to chair the State Medical Society's Committee on Obstetrics in 1890. State Medical Society of Wisconsin, "Officers and Members," *Transactions* 24 (1890–1891): x.

76. See Milwaukee Health Department, Physicians' Register, January 10, 1888. Klaes had trained with Dr. Graettinger, probably at the Wisconsin College of Midwifery, for she listed her graduation date as 1888.

77. Advertisement for the Wisconsin College of Midwifery in Wright's *Milwaukee City Directory* (Milwaukee: Alfred G. Wright, 1896), p. 1093.

78. "City Brevities" in the *Milwaukee Sentinel,* July 2, 1889, p. 3, noted the filing of Articles of Incorporation for the Wisconsin College of Midwifery on July 1, 1889. H. Junge, A. W. Traverse, Louis Berg, Mary Klaes, and Carrie Beckerie were listed as the incorporators.

79. Using the Milwaukee Health Department midwife file, the advertisements in the Milwaukee city directories, and the state licenses, I identified eleven physicians associated with the Wisconsin College of Midwifery between 1885 and 1913, all regular practitioners. Eight of the eleven were American-educated. The mean number of years out of medical school for the eleven was 4.63, with a standard deviation of 3.89. Therefore, if each man was about 23 years old upon graduation from medical school, he was about 28 years old when he began his association with the Wisconsin College of Midwifery.

80. The street listings for Milwaukee in the 1900 manuscript U.S. Census listed Mary Klaes of 318 Cherry Street as the head of the household. The building housed not only the school and the associated lying-in hospital, but also Klaes's daughter, her grandson, and one male and eleven female boarders. The female boarders may

have been unmarried mothers who were patients in her lying-in hospital, for most of them were women in their late teens and early twenties. U.S. Department of Commerce, Bureau of the Census, *Twelfth Census of the United States, 1900,* Manuscript Schedule, Milwaukee, Wisconsin (microfilm). An ad for the school in Wright's *Milwaukee City Directory* for 1897 supports this hypothesis. The text urged physicians "knowing respectable families wishing to adopt a child to call or write the school." *Milwaukee City Directory* (Milwaukee: Alfred G. Wright, 1897), "Lying-In Hospitals," p. 1126.

81. See, for example, state license applications of Rosina Zoladkiewitz and Hattie Tomzak, who graduated in 1912 (Midwife Licenses, WSHS).

82. Wright's *Milwaukee City Directory* (1893), advertisement under "Lying-In Hospitals," p. 1178. Midwives were never mentioned.

83. Wright's *Milwaukee City Directory* (Milwaukee: Alfred G. Wright, 1901), advertisement under "Hospitals," p. 1262.

84. License applications of Caroline Fuss and Maria Timm, Midwife File, WSHS.

85. The city directory advertisements for the lying-in hospital indicate that, like Mrs. Stein's hospital, Klaes's was meant to appeal mainly to unwed mothers looking for a circumspect place to deliver their babies. The copy, for example, advised those wishing to adopt a baby to inquire at the hospital. However, it appears that attempts to combine discretion with education were not always successful, especially for the parturient women involved. A city directory advertisement for a third lying-in hospital, also run by a midwife, noted in large letters that it was "strictly private" and that clients would not be "annoyed by students." Advertisement for "The Only Local Private Institute for Ladies" under "Lying-In Hospitals," Wright's *Milwaukee City Directory* (1892), p. 1088. This advertisement ran alongside the ones for the other two schools in the city directories throughout the 1890s.

86. Two 1913 graduates of the school, Stefonia Staigwillo and Gertrude Turzynski, noted on their state license applications that they had attended the "full course" of the Wisconsin College of Midwifery. The full course was described as an eight-month term from September to May with hospital time and attendance at twenty-five cases (Midwife File, WSHS).

87. J. Whitridge Williams, "Medical Education and the Midwife Problem in the United States," *Journal of the American Medical Association* 58 (1912): 1–7. Williams found that the general attitude towards obstetrics teaching to be "a very dark spot in our system of medical education" (p. 1).

88. Illinois State Board of Health, *Annual Report* 19 (1896): cii–ciii; cited by Mary Elizabeth Fiorenza, "Midwifery and the Law in Illinois and Wisconsin, 1877–1917" (master's thesis, University of Wisconsin—Madison, 1985), p. 45.

89. Perry, "Early Midwives of Missouri," p. 16.

90. Stein was sixty-one in 1900; her school folded after 1904. Klaes was sixty-two in 1910; the last students of her school graduated in 1913.

91. Kosmak, "Results of Supervised Midwife Practice in Certain European Countries," p. 2009.

92. Edgar, "Education, Licensing, and Supervision of the Midwife," pp. 394–395.

93. "Catalog of the St. Louis School of Midwives," *St. Louis Clinical Record* 2 (1875), advertisement section, pages unnumbered. Quoted by Perry, "Early Midwives of Missouri," p. 16.

94. The 1909 Wisconsin statute licensing midwives was part of the Medical Practice

Act. The physician-controlled Board of Medical Examiners reviewed each application and administered an examination that physicians had written. State of Wisconsin, Statutes, ch. 528 §1435f (1909). In contrast to the complete control over midwife practice, the Board's committee for masseurs appointed the president and the secretary of the Wisconsin Association of Masseurs and Masseuses to "assist in the examination of applications for registration" (State Board of Medical Examiners, Minutes 1915–1945, "Minutes for January 11, 1916," Series 1603, Archives Division, State Historical Society of Wisconsin).

95. In an early 1970s study of midwives in history, Barbara Ehrenreich and Deirdre English attributed the decline of midwives in the United States to the sexism and the growing elitism of the American medical profession. See their *Witches, Midwives, and Nurses: A History of Women Healers* (New York: The Feminist Press, 1973), esp. p. 28.

96. Florence Swift Wright, "The Unlicensed Midwife," *Public Health Nurse* 11 (1919): 719.

97. License application of Ida Hill, Tomah, Wisconsin, Midwife File, WSHS.

98. License of Clara Bogenschild, Midwife File, WSHS.

99. Reports of midwifery activity around the United States noted that some midwives were doing obstetrical care. Huntington, in his study of Massachusetts, for example, noted, "Little can be said about the Russian midwives except that they do very little work, nearly all of the five practicing now solely as obstetrical nurses" ("Midwives in Massachusetts," p. 544).

100. Melosh points out that private duty nurses faced the same problem in the 1920s, ultimately losing much of their autonomy when they went back to the hospital as staff nurses. "The organization of private duty locked nurses into relationships of personal service: physicians' authority and patients' caprices interfered with nurses' ability to define their own work" (Melosh, *"The Physician's Hand,"* p. 82).

2. A Married Woman's Occupation

1. License application of Dora Larson, Board of Medical Examiners, Midwife File, Series 1611, Archives Division, Wisconsin State Historical Society (hereafter Midwife File, WSHS). Personal data on Dora Larson were obtained from the manuscript census of 1910, Wiota Township, Lafayette County. U.S. Department of Commerce, Bureau of the Census, *Twelfth Census of the United States, 1900,* Manuscript Schedule, Lafayette County, Wisconsin (microfilm).

2. Data on Emilie Roller came from the manuscript portion of the 1880 census and from her license application with the state. U.S. Department of Commerce, Bureau of the Census, *Tenth Census of the United States, 1880,* Manuscript Schedule, Milwaukee, Wisconsin, (microfilm); license application of Emilie Roller, Midwife File, WSHS. Roller trained at the Kaiseren Louise Midwifery School in Posen, Germany, graduating in 1872. She was practicing in Milwaukee by 1880, and she continued to attend birthing women into the twentieth century. Roller and Larson were two of the 398 midwives identified either through the Milwaukee Health Department Registry, the State License Files, or the Milwaukee City Directory whom I traced to the federal manuscript census schedules of either 1880, 1900, or 1910 or the Wisconsin state census of 1905.

3. Frances E. Kobrin, in her pioneering article on midwives, described the decline of midwifery in the early twentieth century as due to a problem of professionalization within the medical profession. See Frances E. Kobrin, "The American Midwife Controversy: A Crisis of Professionalization," *Bulletin of the History of Medicine* 40 (1966): 350–363. I argue that midwifery itself faced a "crisis of professionalization," based on the nature of the practitioner and how midwifery was practiced.

4. Regina Markell Morantz-Sanchez, *Sympathy and Science: Women Physicians in American Medicine* (New York: Oxford University Press, 1985), p. 93.

5. Mary Roth Walsh notes that the costs of medical school rose throughout the nineteenth century and that most medical students as early as the 1860s were the daughters of well-off families. See Walsh, *"Doctors Wanted: No Women Need Apply": Sexual Barriers in the Medical Profession, 1835–1975* (New Haven: Yale University Press, 1977), p. 62.

6. Dr. Emily Pope's 1881 survey of 430 female doctors found that 15.1 percent of the respondents had married and 78 percent of the married doctors continued to practice. Emily F. Pope, "The Practice of Medicine by Women in the United States," *Journal of Social Science* 13 (March 1881): 8. This trend had changed by 1900. Regina Morantz-Sanchez and Gloria Moldow both found that about one-third female physicians were married either before starting school or after finishing school. See Morantz-Sanchez, *Sympathy and Science,* p. 107, no. 127, and Gloria Moldow, *Women Doctors in Gilded-Age Washington* (Urbana: University of Illinois Press, 1987), p. 34. By 1939, a survey of Wellesley College graduates who had gone into medicine revealed a much larger percentage of married women doctors. Of the Wellesley doctors, 42 percent had married, and about 75 percent of these married doctors had had children. Most of these physicians continued to practice. Alice Ames Kavanagh, Edith Midwood Perrin, and Jean Watt Gorely, "Wellesley in Medicine," *Wellesley Magazine* (March 1939): 288.

7. Nancy Tomes, " 'Little World of Our Own': The Pennsylvania Hospital Training School for Nurses, 1895–1907," in Judith Walzer Leavitt, ed., *Women and Health in America: Historical Readings,* (Madison: University of Wisconsin Press, 1984), pp. 467–481. At the Johns Hopkins Nursing School, most of the students were Protestant, well educated, and usually not self-supporting. Indeed, this background seemed to be required, as nursing students were chosen on the basis of their "refinement" by the professionally minded superintendent, Isabel Hampton. See Janet Wilson James, "Isabel Hampton and the Professionalization of Nursing in the 1890s," in Morris J. Vogel and Charles E. Rosenberg, eds., *The Therapeutic Revolution: Essays in the Social History of Medicine* (Philadelphia: University of Pennsylvania Press, 1979), pp. 201–244.

8. Barbara Melosh, *"The Physician's Hand:" Work Culture and Conflict in American Nursing* (Philadelphia: Temple University Press, 1982), p. 10.

9. Susan M. Reverby, *Ordered to Care: The Dilemma of American Nursing, 1850–1945,* Cambridge History of Medicine (New York: Cambridge University Press, 1987), p. 213, Table A7.

10. Reverby notes that graduates of the nursing school of the Boston city asylum, for example, were told bluntly by physicians and directors of nurse registries that they could not expect to receive the same wages as graduates of the "better schools" of nursing in Boston, who were usually women of higher social status. See Reverby, " 'Neither for the Drawing Room nor for the Kitchen': Private Duty

Nursing in Boston, 1873–1920," in Leavitt, *Women and Health in America,* pp. 454–466.

11. See Tomes, " 'Little World of Our Own,' " for a discussion of how the director of the Pennsylvania Hospital School, Lucy Walker, sought to create a disciplined, reliable, well-mannered nurse who, at the very least, could be depended upon to make "a fine private duty nurse for a middle-class family" (p. 477).

12. Reverby, *Ordered to Care,* pp. 111–112. Reverby points out, however, that like other professional women, many nurses never married (p. 112).

13. Dorothy and Richard Wertz, in *Lying In: A History of Childbirth in America* (New York: Schocken Books, 1977), coined the term "social childbirth" to describe the almost exclusively female network of family and friends who would gather to help early American women through the ordeal of childbirth. Judith Walzer Leavitt, in *Brought to Bed: Childbearing in America, 1750–1950* (New York: Oxford University Press, 1986), further developed the idea of social childbirth, arguing that throughout the nineteenth century, women who gave birth at home continued to ask family and friends to assist them, and that the sex of the birth attendant was immaterial.

14. Nursing was not considered compatible with the demands of family life because private duty nursing, the usual job nurses assumed after graduation, often involved twenty-four-hour, around-the-clock care for a patient in the patient's home. See Susan Reverby, " 'Neither for the Drawing Room nor for the Kitchen.' "

15. Several feminist theorists have explored the gender differences of personality development over the life cycle. These differences, they argue, help to explain why women's personalities tend to be defined in terms of relation and connection to other people, rather than the more masculine ideal of hierarchy and individual achievement. Using Freudian object-relations theory, Nancy Chodorow traces this personality development to the fact that women universally are responsible for child care. The psychological result of this arrangement is that girls, identifying with their mothers, come to see themselves as much more connected to others, and so acquire a basis of empathy. Exploring the moral development of women, Carol Gilligan traces this idea through the life cycle, arguing that women throughout their lives continue to place greater importance on attachment than on separation, autonomy, individuation, or natural rights. See Nancy Chodorow, *The Reproduction of Mothering: Psychoanalysis and the Sociology of Gender* (Berkeley: University of California Press, 1978); and Carol Gilligan, *In a Different Voice: Psychological Theory and Women's Development* (Cambridge: Harvard University Press, 1982). While it is impossible to psychologically analyze the motivations of people in the past, these theories of gender suggest some underlying reasons why married, immigrant midwives might not have even considered the need to professionalize their occupation. Childbirth with a midwife had always been a social affair, where the midwife was part of a team of women assisting the birthing mother. As Chapters 3 and 4 show, the majority of midwives cared for women of their own ethnic group, perhaps reinforcing the belief that caring and empathy were as important as the technical skills of midwifery. In many ways, nurses faced a similar obstacle to professionalization. As Susan Reverby notes, nursing is an occupation charged with the obligation to care, and care was defined as women's work (Reverby, *Ordered to Care,* pp. 1–7).

16. See the appendix for a discussion of the sample techniques on how these midwives were chosen. The midwife families were found in either the 1870, the 1880, the 1900, or the 1910 federal manuscript census schedules or in the 1905 Wisconsin state

manuscript census. As the appendix notes, of the 893 different midwives in the fifty-year period of my study (1870–1920), I was able to link 398 (43.4 percent) to the census.

17. "Figures that Don't Lie," *Milwaukee Sentinel,* June 23, 1889, p. 12.

18. The source of my data is the listings under "Midwife" in the classified ad section of Wright's *Milwaukee City Directory.* I sampled the directories for five-year periods beginning in 1870 and ending in 1930. The first year a woman advertised I considered her cohort year, and each woman in a cohort was followed in succeeding directories. City directories are not definitive sources for locating people in the late nineteenth and early twentieth centuries, especially those such as midwives, who came from working-class, ethnic backgrounds. Thus, small changes may not be significant, but large changes in the numbers of midwives, as shown in Figure 2.1, may be. For a discussion of the sources used in this and the succeeding chapters, see the appendix.

19. Kobrin, "The American Midwife Controversy"; also Jane Pacht Brickman, "Public Health, Midwives, and Nurses, 1880–1930," in Ellen Condliffe Lagemann, ed., *Nursing History: New Perspectives, New Possibilities* (New York: Teacher's College Press, 1983), p. 70; Elizabeth Ewen, *Immigrant Women in the Land of Dollars: Life and Culture on the Lower East Side, 1890–1925* (New York: Monthly Review Press, 1985), p. 130; Eugene Declerq, "The Nature and Style of Practice of Immigrant Midwives in Early Twentieth-Century Massachusetts," *Journal of Social History* 19 (1985): 115. Declerq's Table 2, p. 117, shows that all of the "major midwives" in Lawrence were born in Europe.

20. Michael M. Davis, *Immigrant Health and the Community* (New York: Harper and Brothers, 1921), p. 195.

21. Florence S. Wright, "The Midwives and Our Foreign Born in America," *Public Health Nurse* 11 (1919): 661.

22. Joseph B. DeLee, "Progress toward Ideal Obstetrics," *American Journal of Obstetrics and Diseases of Women and Children* 73 (1916): 412.

23. Arthur Brewster Emmons and James Lincoln Huntington, "Has the Trained and Supervised Midwife Made Good?" *Transactions for the American Association for the Study and the Prevention of Infant Mortality* 2 (1911): 209; Huntington, "Midwifery in Massachusetts," *Boston Medical and Surgical Journal* 167 (1912).

24. Befitting the immigrant history of Minnesota, over one-third of the midwives were from Scandinavian counties; 17.1 percent were German. E. C. Hartley and Ruth E. Boynton, "A Survey of the Midwife Situation in Minnesota," *Minnesota Medicine* 7 (1924): 441, Table 3.

25. Florence Brown Sherbon and Elizabeth Moore, *Maternity and Infant Care in Two Rural Counties in Wisconsin,* U.S. Department of Labor, Children's Bureau Publication no. 46 (Washington, D.C.: Government Printing Office, 1919), p. 10.

26. Ibid., pp. 30–32.

27. Expected numbers were derived from a chi-square analysis of county by birthplace. The results were highly significant; the chi-square = 207.949, significant at 0.00001. The three rural counties had many more Scandinavian midwives than would be expected, and Milwaukee city had many fewer (Milwaukee had only 4 Scandinavian midwives, 37.1 expected). Price and Trempealeau counties also had many fewer German birth attendants than would be expected (Trempealeau had no German midwives, 13.9 were expected; Price had 8 instead of 20.3).

28. Neal Devitt, citing the results of six important early twentieth-century midwife

studies, concluded that the majority of midwives in the northern United States were literate, over thirty-five years old, and foreign-born. Going further, he argued that "the advanced age of most midwives and their immigrant origins . . . play[ed] a crucial role in their elimination." Neal Devitt, "The Statistical Case for Elimination of the Midwife: Fact versus Prejudice, 1890–1935," Part 1, *Women and Health* 4, 1 (Spring 1979): 84]. See also Josephine Baker's study of New York City ("Schools for Midwives," *Transactions of the American Association for the Study and Prevention of Infant Mortality* 2 [1911]: 232–248), F. Elisabeth Crowell's 1908 study of Chicago ("The Midwives of Chicago," *Journal of the American Medical Association* 50 [1908]: 1346–1350), Mary Sherwood's 1909 analysis of Baltimore ("The Midwives of Baltimore," *Journal of the American Medical Association* 52 [1909]: 2009–2011), and Louis Schultz Reed's 1932 examination of midwives in Minnesota, New Jersey, and Texas *Midwives, Chiropodists, and Optometrists, Their Place in Medical Care* [Washington, D.c.: The Committee on the Costs of Medical Care, 1932]).

29. Agnes C. Vietor, ed., *A Woman's Quest: The Life of Marie Zakrzewska, M.D.* (New York: D. Appleton, 1924), p. 39. Zakrzewska was eighteen years old when she first sought admission to the Midwifery School of Berlin. Eventually, through the entreaties of a powerful friend, the physician of the King of Prussia, she was admitted to the school (pp. 39–42).

30. The mean age of all of the respondents was 48.05, with a standard deviation of 12.38 (Midwife File, WSHS). A one-way ANOVA showed significant differences, with an F-value of 7.725, $p = 0.00001$.

31. A one-way ANOVA showed no significant differences between groups of midwives identified in any of the five census years (f-ratio $= 1.28$, with an insignificant of 0.2776).

32. The standard deviation from the mean for married midwives in this sample was 9.93. The mean age of the eleven divorced women, 42.64, was similar to that of the married women. The standard deviation for divorced midwives was 12.23. A one-way analysis of variance showed significant differences between these groups: the f-ratio between groups was 16.92, significant at the 0.01 level. A Scheffe procedure was run to test significant differences between pairs of groups. The mean age of the widows was significantly higher than that of the single or married midwives, and the age of the married practitioners was significantly higher than that of the single ones (at the 0.05 level).

33. Joan W. Scott and Louise A. Tilly, "Women's Work and the Family in Nineteenth-Century Europe," *Comparative Studies in Society and History* 17 (1975): 40.

34. Elizabeth H. Pleck found that few immigrant married women worked for wages outside of the home. See "A Mother's Wages: Income Earning among Married Italian and Black Women, 1896–1911," in Michael Gordon, ed., *The American Family in Social-Historical Perspective,* 2d ed. (New York: St. Martin's Press, 1978), p. 492. Leslie Woodcock Tentler found that only 5.6 percent of all married women were reported to be at work outside the home, in 1900. See Tentler, *Wage-Earning Women: Industrial Work and Family Life in the United States, 1900–1930* (New York: Oxford University Press, 1979), p. 137.

35. For an analysis of the strong relationship between midwifery and the other aspects of women's traditional domestic responsibilities in a preindustrial economy, see Laurel Thatcher Ulrich, *A Midwife's Tale: The Life of Martha Ballard, Based on Her Diary, 1785–1812* (New York: Alfred A. Knopf, 1990).

36. To code for husbands' occupation, I used the categories defined by the federal census of 1940. The categories are roughly hierarchical, except for the two categories in the middle defining farming and mining. To approximate white collar versus blue collar occupations, I grouped the professional, managerial, clerical, and sales categories into one group and the transport, artisan, service, and laborer categories into another. Only 39 midwife husbands fell into the white collar group (12.4 percent), while 201 husbands (64.01 percent) were clearly blue collar. The farm husbands, all located in the three rural counties, were hard to categorize, as farm values varied tremendously.

37. A chi-square analysis of midwives' birthplace by husbands' occupation was highly significant: the $X^2 = 130.85$, with 15 *df,* significant at 0.00001.

38. On the intersection of housework and the marketplace in nineteenth-century America, see, for example, Ruth Schwartz Cowan, *More Work for Mother: The Ironies of Household Technology from the Open Hearth to the Microwave* (New York: Basic Books, 1983); Susan Strasser, *Never Done: A History of American Housework* (New York: Pantheon Books, 1982); Dana Frank, "Housewives, Socialists, and the Politics of Food: The 1917 New York Cost-of-Living Protests," *Feminist Studies* 11 (Summer 1985): 255–285; Elizabeth Ewen, *Immigrant Women in the Land of Dollars;* for Europe, Scott and Tilly, "Women's Work and the Family in Nineteenth-Century Europe," remains a standard reference.

39. Leslie Tentler, *Wage-Earning Women,* pp. 137–138. Thus, of the 20 percent of women who were reported to be working, only half (or 10 percent of the total sample) actually worked outside the home.

40. John Modell and Tamara K. Hareven, "Urbanization and the Malleable Household: An Examination of Boarding and Lodging in American Families," *Journal of Marriage and the Family* 35 (1973): 467–479. See p. 473 for a discussion of the implications of boarding for women's work in the home.

41. Pleck, "A Mother's Wages," p. 497. Louise Lamphere's study of working women who lived in the area around Central Falls, Rhode Island, found that Polish mothers in particular took in boarders: 49 of her 74 sampled Polish households had boarders. Louise Lamphere, *From Working Daughters to Working Mothers: Immigrant Women in a New England Industrial Community* (Ithaca: Cornell University Press, 1987), p. 157.

42. A chi-square analysis of midwives' birthplace by the type of household showed no significant differences ($X^2 = 22.98$, with 20 *df, p* = 0.2896); the same was true of a chi-square analysis of husbands' occupation by the type of household ($X^2 = 16.409$, *df* = 12, *p* = 0.1732—insignificant).

43. Modell and Hareven, "Urbanization and the Malleable Household," pp. 471–473.

44. Information on children was obtained for 387 women. The mean number of children was 2.99, with a standard deviation of 2.41.

45. An analysis of variance showed no significant differences between groups. The *f*-ratio was 0.99 and the *f*-probability equaled 0.37.

46. Lynn Y. Weiner points out that children after this age had the potential to replace and then make more money than their mothers. See Weiner, *From Working Girl to Working Mother: The Female Labor Force in the United States, 1820–1920* (Chapel Hill: University of North Carolina Press, 1985), p. 85.

47. The median age of oldest children of all midwives was fifteen, with a modal

(most frequent number) age of nine. However, the range of ages was quite broad, from one to fifty-four years.

48. In order to analyze the number of births attended by each practitioner or group of practitioners, the births file was sorted and aggregated by county, attendant number, and attendant status. A new variable, "NBABES," captured the total number of babies overseen by each doctor or midwife. Matching the midwives in this file to the census data by linking the attendant numbers, the resulting file had information on 274 midwives. I performed a stepwise multiple regression, with number of babies as the dependent variable. The number of children, age of the oldest, age of the youngest, and the midwife's own age were entered as independent variables. Only age of the midwife had an F-value significant enough to enter into the regression equation ($F = 7.101$, significance $= 0.0082$). The resultant R^2 equaled 0.02194, showing that age only very weakly explained the total number of babies delivered.

49. Stephan Thernstrom, *Poverty and Progress: Social Mobility in a Nineteenth-Century City* (Cambridge: Harvard University Press, 1964), pp. 121–122, 129–130; also Ronald Tobey, Charles Wetherell, and Jay Brigham, "Moving Out and Settling In: Residential Mobility, Home Owning, and the Public Enframing of Citizenship, 1921–1950," *American Historical Review* 95 (1990): 1395–1422. These authors argue that the long-term mortgage was responsible for expanding opportunities for home ownership, which then restrained America's historic mobility. In the 1920s, most home mortgages had terms averaging from five to ten years, and three-year mortgages were not unheard of. The development of FHA mortgages in the 1930s, they point out, doubled the average term of a household mortgage from less than ten years to twenty years.

50. Thernstrom, *Poverty and Progress,* pp. 120–121. There were a few differences in the status of the home when the birthplace of the midwife was considered. Many more Scandinavians than expected owned their homes outright (20 actual versus 8.3 expected). Polish midwife families, which tended to be laborers' families, had higher than expected numbers of renters (25 versus 17.6 expected), and lower than expected numbers of home owners (5 versus 8.7 expected). However, they also had higher than expected numbers of families holding mortgages (15 actual versus only 11 expected). $X^2 = 56.42$, $df = 15$, significant at 0.00001.

51. One-way ANOVAs were used to test whether the size of a midwife's practice was related to her socioeconomic status. For husbands' occupation, the f-ratio was 1.3700, with 7 df, and an f-probability of 0.2202. For home status, the f-ratio was 1.7649, with 2 df, and an f-probability of 0.1736. One explanation of this lack of difference in home ownership and in family structure between different classes of midwife families may be that the distance between artisan wages and those of unskilled laborers may not have been very large. Indeed, the Wisconsin data suggest that the financial struggles of artisan families may have been greater than those of day laborers. The problems faced by midwife artisan families were revealed by a chi-square analysis of occupation and home ownership. When midwife husbands' occupations were cross-tabulated by home ownership, instead of artisan families predominantly owning their homes and laborers mostly renting, more artisan families than expected rented and fewer of them owned houses outright than would be expected. On the other hand, fewer laborers' families rented and more of them had mortgaged or fully owned homes than would be expected. Of interest was the high degree of home ownership among farmers: only 4 midwife farm families rented their homes.

(Chi-square was significant: $X^2 = 50.098$, 9 df, significant at 0.0001. A study of the wages of both skilled and unskilled immigrant groups in Iowa at the end of the nineteenth century suggests that the difference in income between skilled and unskilled immigrant workers was not as significant as previously thought. Immigrants with previous knowledge of a trade earned more at first than immigrants without training. However, unskilled immigrants managed subsequently to close some of the gap by rapid advancement on the job. See Barry Eichengreen and Henry A. Gemery, "The Earnings of Skilled and Unskilled Immigrants at the End of the Nineteenth Century," *Journal of Economic History* 46 (1986): 441–454.

52. Density of population undoubtedly played some part in determining the size of a practice for a rural or an urban midwife, just as it did for physician practice. A study done by the American Medical Association in 1917 reported that the greatest number of physicians lived not in the nation's largest cities, but in small towns with populations between 2,500 and 10,000. Physicians who lived in these towns also served the rural areas. Even so, in rural areas there was only one doctor for every 991 persons. In addition, the problems of transportation in rural areas undoubtedly circumscribed the size of a birth attendant's practice. Committee on Social Insurance, *Statistics Regarding the Medical Profession,* Social Insurance Series Pamphlet no. 7 (Chicago: American Medical Association [1917]), pp. 11, 19–20; cited by Ronald L. Numbers, *Almost Persuaded: American Physicians and Compulsory Health Insurance, 1912–1920,* Henry E. Sigerist Supplement, *Bulletin of the History of Medicine,* new series, no. 1 (Baltimore: The Johns Hopkins University Press, 1978), p. 4.

53. Rudolph Holmes et al., "The Midwives of Chicago, Being a Report of a Joint Committee of the Chicago Medical Society and Hull House," *Journal of the American Medical Association* 51 (1908): 1348.

54. Huntington, "Midwives in Massachusetts," p. 544.

3. Neighbor Women in the Country

1. Florence Brown Sherbon and Elizabeth Moore, *Maternity and Infant Care in Two Rural Counties in Wisconsin,* U.S. Department of Labor, Children's Bureau Publication no. 46 (Washington, D.C.: Government Printing Office, 1919), p. 13.

2. Ibid., p. 32.

3. Biographical information is from the 1900 United States manuscript census for Trempealeau County. U.S. Department of Commerce, Bureau of the Census, *Twelfth Census of the United States, 1900,* Manuscript Schedule, Trempealeau County, Wisconsin (microfilm). Folkedahl's husband was reported as a "laborer"; presumably, in this heavily agricultural county, he was a farm laborer. Training information on Anna Folkedahl was obtained from her state midwifery license application. [Board of Medical Examiners, Midwife File, Series 1611, Archives Division, Wisconsin State Historical Society, Madison, Wisconsin (hereafter referred to as Midwife File, WSHS).

4. The birth record for Schiedt recorded that the attendant was the mother-in-law of the parturient. Birth Records, Dane County, Wisconsin, May 5, 1900. Filed with Dane County Vital Records Office, City-County Building, Madison, Wisconsin (hereafter referred to as Birth Records, Dane County, DCVRO).

5. The numbers of births were averaged over a year. The number of deliveries is not a continuous variable; its distribution is not a normal distribution, and thus it is

likely to be affected by different variances and nonnormal distributions. This, in turn, means that the error terms would also be distributed as nonnormal. However, number of deliveries was a proven, crucial variable, so I proceeded with tests of significance. For a further discussion of the problems with this type of distribution, see the appendix.

6. Sherbon and Moore, *Maternity and Infant Care,* pp. 13, 33.

7. In 1910, about 14 percent of farms in the state were operated by tenants. Sherbon and Moore, *Maternity and Infant Care,* p. 57.

8. John Mack Faragher points out that despite the cultural idea of gender-divided "separate spheres" in the nineteenth century, the vast majority of rural women lived with men in families. See Faragher, *Women and Men on the Overland Trail* (New Haven: Yale University Press, 1979), pp. 1–2. Nancy Grey Osterud ties this relationship to economic reality: rural women, she argues, could not support themselves outside of a male-headed farm household. Osterud, *Bonds of Community: The Lives of Farm Women in Nineteenth-Century New York* (Ithaca: Cornell University Press, 1991), p. 2.

9. For a detailed history of the development of agricultural practices in Wisconsin, see Robert C. Nesbit, *Wisconsin: A History* (Madison: University of Wisconsin Press, 1973). Chapter 19, "King Wheat Dethroned" (pp. 280–295), and Chapter 20, "Empire in Pine" (pp. 296–312), are especially relevant to understanding the economies of Trempealeau and Price Counties. Information on farms in Price County can be found in the Agricultural Experiment Station and Agricultural Extension Service's *Story of Price County, Wisconsin: Population Research in a Rural Development County* (Research Bulletin 220, University of Wisconsin, Madison, June 1960), p. 10. The number of farms increased each decade as follows:

1880	42
1890	380
1900	885
1910	1,352
1920	1,935

10. Sherbon and Moore's study of childbearing conditions in two Wisconsin counties in 1916 *(Maternity and Infant Care)* found that many mothers sold cream and made butter from their dairy farms. Some Polish women in Marathon County, they found, even cut cordwood to earn money to pay for the groceries (pp. 44–45). A Children's Bureau study of rural Montana found that farm women's sale of butter enabled their families to purchase necessary improvements such as windmills. Viola Paradise, *Maternity Care and the Welfare of Young Children in a Homesteading County in Montana,* U.S. Department of Labor, Children's Bureau, Rural Child Welfare Series no. 3 (Washington, D.C.: Government Printing Office, 1919), p. 14. Nancy Grey Osterud argues that "the gender division of labor intersected with capitalist expansion to produce substantial asymmetries in men's and women's relationship to the market." While men were producing grain and other products for more distant markets, women continued to sell small quantities of eggs and other products that yielded petty cash for the household. Osterud, *Bonds of Community,* pp. 209–211.

11. See Osterud, *Bonds of Community,* Chapter 9, "Value of Women's Work," pp. 202–227.

12. In the three counties, 139 "rural" midwives were identified from the sampled birth records. All midwives in Trempealeau and Price Counties were considered rural

midwives; in Dane County, midwives who lived in the city of Madison were excluded. Of the 139 total, 72 delivered only one baby. The numbers for each county were as follows:

County	Total no. midwives	Single-birth midwives	Ratio
Trempealeau	45	20	.444
Price	61	33	.541
Dane (rural)	33	17	.515

13. Sherbon and Moore, *Maternity and Infant Care,* p. 34. Mrs. R. reportedly never had a doctor's assistance at any of her own births, and sometimes she did not even have the assistance of a neighbor. As a neighborhood midwife, she was not known to charge a fee, but her neighbors "just gave her something," generally about $2 to $3.

14. Birth record of Sandven, December 18, 1910, Birth Records, Dane County, DCVRO. Mrs. Renz was not found to have attended another birth. Very few of the midwives in the three counties who attended only one birth left their own villages. Of the seventeen midwives in Dane County who delivered only one baby, all were from the same village as the mother. In Trempealeau County, two neighbor-woman midwives traveled to the next village, and in Price County, three of the neighbor women left their own villages.

15. Judith Walzer Leavitt notes that the options throughout the nineteenth century for rural childbearing women were limited. She found that significant numbers of women reported that they delivered their own babies or enlisted the help of their husbands. See Judith Walzer Leavitt, *Brought to Bed: Childbearing in America, 1750–1950* (New York: Oxford University Press, 1986), p. 79.

16. To check on the location of midwife practice, I compared the location of the midwife to the location of the birth that she attended. No neighbor-woman midwife in Dane County left her village; four midwives each probably left their village in Trempealeau and Price Counties. One of the Trempealeau County midwives was a Minnesota midwife who came across the Mississippi River to attend a birth in the riverfront town of Trempealeau.

17. Osterud, *Bonds of Community,* p. 117.

18. Glenn Steele, *Maternity and Infant Care in a Mountain County in Georgia,* U.S. Department of Labor, Children's Bureau Publication no. 120 (Washington, D.C.: Government Printing Office, 1923), p. 16. Unlike some southern areas studied by the Children's Bureau, the population of this county appears to have been all white (pp. 2–3).

19. Paradise, *Maternity Care,* p. 31. This Montana study found that few female birth attendants had attended more than one or two births per year in the preceding year. A few of these women had been trained as practical nurses, and they reported that they preferred to work with physicians (p. 32).

20. In Marathon County, for example, of fourteen midwives from whom information about training could be obtained, two had attended a training school and several more had been taught by physicians. Sherbon and Moore, *Maternity and Infant Care,* pp. 30–31.

21. Training information for Folkedahl, Semerau, and the Price and Trempealeau

apprentice-trained midwives is from Midwife File, WSHS. Ottile Lange registered with the Milwaukee Health Department in 1881, before she moved to Wauwatosa (Physicians' Register, City of Milwaukee Health Department, Archives Section, Milwaukee Public Library, Milwaukee, Wisconsin, hereafter known as Milwaukee Health Department, Physicians' Register).

22. See midwife license application for Mrs. Charles Hjort, Midwife File, WSHS. The births attended by Mrs. Hjort were from Birth Records, Price County, Wisconsin. Filed with State of Wisconsin Department of Health and Human Services Vital Records Office, Madison, Wisconsin (hereafter known as Birth Records, Price County, WSHS).

23. Larson went out only once in 1900, the first year she appeared in the sample, but in 1905 she attended seventeen births and in 1910 she oversaw fifteen. By 1915 her practice had shrunk to five births, and in 1920 she went out only once. Cases tabulated from the Birth Records for Trempealeau and Price Counties. Trempealeau County records were filed at the State of Wisconsin Department of Health and Human Services Vital Records Office, Madison, Wisconsin (hereafter known as Birth Records, Trempealeau County, WSHS). Like Larson, many rural midwives started with a few deliveries and then had one or two sample years when they attended a significant number. Their practices then declined until they stopped practicing entirely.

24. Price County was organized as a separate county in 1885. Rachel Berry was probably practicing midwifery before this date. However, I did not find her practicing at all after 1886.

25. Sherbon and Moore, *Maternity and Infant Care,* pp. 31–32.

26. Sherbon and Moore, *Maternity and Infant Care,* pp. 21, 27, 59, 61.

27. Osterud, *Bonds of Community,* p. 218.

28. A township in Wisconsin is both a legal and a survey entity. As a legal entity, a township may encompass several villages or cities, and can assess taxes. A township is also a survey object, as each county historically was broken into a certain number of townships. A township covers about thirty-six square miles; it is roughly six miles long on each border. See Sir Dudley Stamp, ed., *Glossary of Geographical Terms* (London: Longman Publishers, 1970), p. 489. The geographic location of midwife practice in Dane County was measured somewhat differently. I divided the county into six concentric circles, with Madison, the most urban place in the county, at the center. Each rural midwife's own home location was compared with the location of the births she attended. Of thirty-nine rural neighbor-woman midwives, twenty-five practiced only in their own sections. Almost all of the remaining fourteen neighbor women went only as far as the two areas contiguous to their own.

29. Larson claimed on her state license to have attended over 4,000 births. However, though she practiced in Trempealeau County at least from 1900 to 1920, she attended only 39 births in the twenty-four total months sampled. This kind of cross-checking led me to doubt the usefulness of the number of cases claimed in the state licenses.

30. Of 21 births sampled in 1905 and 1910, 19 births attended by Folkedahl were in her village of Ettrick.

31. Birth Records, Price County, WSHS; also Manuscript Census for Price County, 1900; and Midwife File, WSHS.

32. Julie Roy Jeffrey notes that women on the frontier called in friends and neigh-

bors to help them. This neighborliness kept childbirth a female-centered event, "with little thought of monetary reward." The birthing woman, however, was expected to provide an adequate amount of prepared food for her women relatives and friends. As one of the frontier women quoted by Jeffrey put it, "There wasn't no paying these friends so you had to treat them good." Jeffrey, *Frontier Women: The Trans-Mississippi West, 1840–1880* (New York: Hill and Wang, 1979), p. 69. In the Children's Bureau study of Montana, one birthing woman gave her two relatives who helped out "a little pig worth $6" (Paradise, *Maternity Care*, p. 51).

33. Sherbon and Moore, *Maternity and Infant Care*, p. 35.

34. Sherbon and Moore, *Maternity and Infant Care*, p. 34. The Montana Children's Bureau study differentiated neighbor women who attended their friends as a favor, without charge, versus women who were called on more regularly for their services. Midwives in this latter group, the researcher reported, "decid[ed] to consider their services as at least professional nursing and [resolved] to charge a fee." The fee ranged from $1.50 to $2.00 per day, to $25.00 per week, which included the price of the delivery. Infrequently, a midwife in this group would charge $25.00 for the delivery alone (Paradise, *Maternity Care*, p. 31).

35. Mrs. M. was described as being "highly esteemed" among her patients, some of whom she had attended many times. Even physicians in this area turned obstetrical care over to Mrs. M. (Sherbon and Moore, *Maternity and Infant Care*, pp. 33–34).

36. The figures are based on computations of the births and the income noted in "Mary Gerrard: Journal of a LaCrosse Midwife," Mss SC 28, Archives Division, University of Wisconsin—LaCrosse Area Research Center, WSHS—LaCrosse. The manuscript is really a birth log and not a journal. My thanks to Jan Coombs for bringing this source to my attention.

37. Butter-making, which remained women's work throughout much of the nineteenth century, provided significant cash to many farm families. Though there is a time lag between the dates of these farm women and Mrs. Gerrard, as Joan Jensen has explained, there are few systematic studies of women's household commodity production. Furthermore, statistics on income from household production were often excluded by census takers. "Cloth, Butter and Boarders: Women's Household Production for the Market," *The Review of Radical Political Economics* 12, 2 (Summer 1980): 14—24.

38. Both Mrs. Nystrum's midwifery license application as well as the birth certificates she filed list her as "Mrs. Rev. John Nystrum." I discovered her given name only through the family's listing in the census. The family details were chronicled in her license application.

39. Rosalind Rosenberg, *Divided Lives: American Women in the Twentieth Century* (New York: Hill and Wang, 1992), p. 11.

40. Mrs. Nystrum reported on her license application that she had attended a total of only twenty births. Julie Roy Jeffrey argues that ministers' wives enjoyed a great deal of respect in their community, even as they labored to raise money for the church and for their own families. Many ministers' wives, she points out, came out to the west expecting to be almost full partners with their husbands in their missionary work (*Frontier Women*, pp. 100–103). In addition, a substantial amount of evidence, dating back to treatises compiled in the seventeenth century, indicates that Protestant congregations expected ministers' wives to be skilled in at least minor medical matters. Several Boston ministers' wives were known for their skill, and Cotton Mather wrote

of the importance of such knowledge, training his own daughter Katy so that she might be of use in distributing medicine to neighbors who came to her in need. Otho T. Beall and Richard Shryock, *Cotton Mather: First Significant Figure in American Medicine* (Baltimore: Johns Hopkins Press, 1954), p. 16. More work is needed on this role for ministers' wives.

41. Sherbon and Moore, *Maternity and Infant Care,* p. 32.

42. U.S. Census, 1880, 1900, 1910; Wisconsin state census, 1905.

43. Sherbon and Moore, *Maternity and Infant Care,* p. 19. By 1900, about 37 percent of the population of Price County was foreign-born, and over 49 percent of these immigrants were from Norway, Sweden, Finland, or Denmark. United States Census, *Twelfth, 1900,* vol. 1, *Population,* pp. 794–795.

44. One-way ANOVA tests of midwives' birthplace and percentages of Scandinavian, German, and American-born patients were highly significant. For all ethnic groups of midwives delivering Scandinavian patients, the f-probability was 0.00001, with an F-ratio of 18.78. A Scheffe test showed significant differences at the 0.05 level. Scandinavian midwives in this test had a mean of 81.75 percent Scandinavian patients. The mean for German midwives was 12.5 percent, and the mean for American midwives was 4.0 percent. Tests for the percentage of German and American-born patients delivered by German and American midwives showed similar results.

45. A chi-square analysis of midwives' birthplace by township was highly significant in Price County. Within each town, there were specific immigrant groups of midwives. The five Finnish midwives, for example, were located only in Knox. Chi-square $=$ 110.34, 48 *df,* significance of 0.00001.

46. Birth records, Price County.

47. Sherbon and Moore, *Maternity and Infant Care,* p. 32.

48. The census study identified five Dane County midwives and six Trempealeau County midwives born in this country. About 55 percent of the patients of Trempealeau County midwives were American, and 29 percent Scandinavian. On the other hand, almost 80 percent of the patients of Dane County American midwives were American-born. In the sampled births over all the years sampled, the average number of babies attended by all the Scandinavian midwives in the three rural areas was 9.32; for the German midwives, the average was 31.43; but the American-born midwives' average was only 4.63.

49. Elizabeth Briggs was the daughter of German immigrants. Sixty-five years old when she applied for a license in 1909, she reported that she had learned midwifery through an apprenticeship (Midwife File, WSHS).

50. Ibid. Of the four Trempealeau County midwives who applied for state licenses, Briggs had by far the smallest practice.

51. Laurel Thatcher Ulrich, *A Midwife's Tale: The Life of Martha Ballard, Based on Her Diary, 1785–1812* (New York: Alfred A. Knopf, 1990), pp. 162–181.

52. See Leavitt, *Brought to Bed;* also Sylvia D. Hoffert, *Private Matters: American Attitudes toward Childbearing and Infant Nurture in the Urban North, 1800–1860* (Urbana: University of Illinois Press, 1989).

4. Midwife Entrepreneurs in the City

1. Details of Mary Gerrard's life were gleaned from several sources. On her training, see Board of Medical Examiners, Midwife File, Series 1611, Archives Divi-

sion, Wisconsin State Historical Society, Madison, Wisconsin (hereafter referred to as Midwife File, WSHS). On her family, see U.S. Department of Commerce, Bureau of the Census, *Twelfth Census of the United States, 1900,* and *Thirteenth Census of the United States, 1910,* Manuscript Schedule, LaCrosse County, Wisconsin (Microfilm); also the Wisconsin State Census, 1905 (microfilm); also obituary notice for Mary Gerrard, "Aged Resident of LaCrosse Dies," *LaCrosse Tribune,* Tuesday, August 24, 1915. My thanks to the staff (especially Michael Edmonds and Lori B. Cook) in the Archives and Microforms Divisions of the Wisconsin State Historical Society for locating this information for me.

2. The 1900 census listed three daughters still at home. Mary, the oldest at nineteen, was not noted as being employed, while seventeen-year-old Bertha was listed as a store clerk. In 1905, however, the three daughters were still living with their parents, as was the Gerrard's son Nicolas, then thirty (Wisconsin State Census, 1905).

3. Wisconsin State Census, 1905. Information on Mary's midwifery practice, which also noted when her family moved to LaCrosse, is found in her birth log, misnamed "Journal." See Mary Gerrard, "Journal of a LaCrosse Midwife," Mss SC 28, University of Wisconsin—LaCrosse Area Research Center, Archives Division, State Historical Society of Wisconsin—LaCrosse. Her birth log noted her charges for each birth as well as the birthdate and sex of the baby. In 1899, she earned $719 for 148 births. In 1904, she earned $564 for 113 births.

4. Michael was listed in the 1905 census as "retired" (Wisconsin State Census, 1905).

5. Gerrard attended an average of about 23 births per year in this period, earning an average of $82.50 per year. She delivered the most babies (36) in 1880, a year in which she was not pregnant. (Gerrard, "Journal").

6. Ibid.

7. As Table 3.1 showed, about 17 percent of urban birth attendants oversaw an average of between one and six deliveries per year, and 32 percent of them attended less than one birth per month on the average. When the number of urban midwives was graphed by their total number of deliveries, I found that 342 midwives attended fewer than forty total deliveries, while 92 attended more than forty. These measures of activity, the average number of births per year and the total number of deliveries in the sample, show that about 20 percent of urban midwives could be considered active, entrepreneurial practitioners.

8. The eighty-eight Milwaukee midwives delivered 6,914 babies out of a total of 10,838 midwife-attended births in Milwaukee County over the period of the sample. The four Madison midwives attended 585 births out of a total of 676.

9. The mean for the Milwaukee midwives was 19.43, and the mean for the Madison midwives was 12.25.

10. Physicians' Register, City of Milwaukee Health Department, Archives Section, Milwaukee Public Library (hereafter Physicians Register, Milwaukee Public Library). See the appendix for a discussion of this source.

11. Roller had overseen at least 700 sampled births by 1909. State of Wisconsin, Department of Health and Human Services, Birth Records, Milwaukee County, Vital Records Office, Madison.

12. Modern lay and nurse-midwives practice, of course, under different circumstances than midwives in the past. However, several types of midwife practitioners have told me that the usual monthly number of home births attended by modern

midwives is about four to six births. A direct-entry midwife (i.e. not a nurse midwife) that a midwife-run clinic in El Paso, Texas, employs six midwives who deliver a total of 90 babies per month (telephone interviews with Deren Bader, midwife in Birmingham, Alabama, January 1993. Physician obstetricians, on the other hand, consider about ten births per month a normal workload. See Martin L. Gonzalez, ed., *Physician Marketplace Statistics, 1992* (Chicago Center for Health Policy Research: American Medical Association, 1992), Table 24, p. 36.

13. Information about the age and family circumstances of Roller and Stange came from the 1880 Federal Manuscript Census. U.S. Department of Commerce, Bureau of the Census, *Tenth Census of the United States, 1880,* Manuscript Schedule, Milwaukee, Wisconsin, (Microfilm). Information on their pace of practice was obtained through an analysis of the birth data from Milwaukee County. Like Emilie Roller, Mary Gerrard reduced the size of her practice after her fiftieth birthday. However, with 90 deliveries, the size of her practice was still large in 1912, the last full year of her practice, when she was sixty-two (Gerrard, "Journal").

14. To assess the possibility of changes over time in the active groups' number of years of practice, in their average age, or in the number of births they attended, I grouped the Milwaukee practitioners into cohorts by the year they first appeared as midwives in the birth records. The eighty-eight midwives formed nine cohorts, spanning the sampled years between 1873 and 1910. (In 1910, only one active midwife began practice, and no active practitioners were found to have begun their practice in 1915 or 1920.) The age of each member of the cohort and the number of deliveries by each member were measured three times: the year the cohort began to practice, the year each member of the cohort reached the peak of her practice, and the year each member quit practice. Thus, a cohort was defined by the year starting practice; however, the years that an individual member of a cohort reached the peak of her practice or left midwifery differed.

15. Cohort membership was determined for each midwife by determining the first year she appeared in the birth records, and the age of each member of each cohort was determined from information found in the census or license records. Each cohort was followed to determine at what age its members reached the zenith of their practice and at what age each member stopped practicing. Because the study was begun at the year 1872, when some midwives were undoubtedly already in practice, birth attendants from the 1872 cohort were considerably older than those in the other cohorts. Therefore, I excluded this cohort from the analysis. Information concerning age was found for 71 of the 90 active Milwaukee midwives. One-way analysis of variance tests of the relationship between age at the beginning of practice, age at the peak of practice, and cohort year showed no significant differences. Similar tests analyzing the relationship between cohort year and number of babies delivered at the beginning of practice, the number of deliveries at the peak of practice, and the number of deliveries at the end of practice showed no significant differences. When census data were brought in, I found that the mean age of the active midwives was 46.9, that 37.0 percent were married to artisans, and that 65.3 percent had three or fewer children living at home (the mean was 2.7). Ages of the children were no different from those reported in the larger census study discussed in Chapter 2. Home ownership could be determined for 47 of these practitioners: 26 (55.3 percent) rented, 12 (25.5 percent) held mortgages, and 9 (19.1 percent) owned their homes outright.

16. Charles V. Chapin, "The Control of Midwifery," in *Children's Bureau, Standards of Child Welfare: A Report of the Children's Bureau Conferences, May and June, 1919,* U.S. Department of Labor, Children's Bureau Publication no. 60 (Washington, D.C.: Government Printing Office, 1919), pp. 158–59.

17. Michael M. Davis, *Immigrant Health and the Community* (New York: Harper and Brothers, 1921), p. 201.

18. Emma Duke, *Infant Mortality: Results of a Field Study in Johnstown, Pennsylvania, Based on Births in One Calendar Year,* U.S. Department of Labor, Children's Bureau Publication no. 9, Infant Mortality Series no. 3 (Washington, D.C.: Government Printing Office, 1915), p. 32.

19. Mary Gerrard's birth log is the only one that I could find for a Wisconsin midwife who practiced during the period under study. It encompasses the years 1878 to 1912. Written in German, each birth is noted with the date, the father's name, the sex of the baby, and the charge for the delivery. Mrs. Gerrard often noted at the end of each year the total number of deliveries that she had attended (Gerrard, "Journal"). LaCrosse was the principal city on the Wisconsin side of the Mississippi River. By the end of the nineteenth century, in fact, it was Wisconsin's "second city." It served as the point where three railroads converged before going on into northern Iowa and Minnesota, and it was also an important lumbering and riverboat-building center. Robert C. Nesbit, *Wisconsin: A History* (Madison: University of Wisconsin Press, 1973), p. 332.

20. The modal (usual) charge for all these years was somewhat higher than the mean charge. As early as 1890, Mary Gerrard's modal charge was $5.00, a figure that did not change until 1907, when it suddenly jumped to $7.00. Throughout all the years of her practice, however, her charges varied from nothing to a high of $10.00, though most of the variations were on the low end. This suggests that she was probably willing to discount her fees somewhat, and that she was less willing to increase them above the usual fee.

21. Though many studies of women's work argue that women (especially single working women) were low paid, it is difficult to find specific numbers. However, Louise Lamphere's study of the textile areas around Central Falls, Rhode Island, gives some wages for 1915. She found that women beyond the entry level were usually paid $9 to $12 per week. Weaving, the most prestigious job for women in the factory, took over a year to learn, but it paid $15 to $18 per week. Louise Lamphere, *From Working Daughters to Working Mothers: Immigrant Women in a New England Industrial Community* (Ithaca: Cornell University Press, 1987), p. 89. Alice Kessler-Harris points out that female wages were always seen as different from male wages. Whatever the value of the product or the productivity of the worker, women's wages would never equal men's. See Alice Kessler-Harris, *A Woman's Wage: Historical Meanings and Social Consequences* (Lexington: University Press of Kentucky, 1990), especially Chapter 1, "The Wage Conceived: Value and Need as Measures of a Woman's Worth," pp. 6–32. Mary Gerrard made nearly as much as John Sedgwick Billings, a young physician in practice in New York City about the same time period. In his first year of practice, in 1897, he reportedly made $520, and he made $684 the next year. By 1899, however, his annual income was over $1,000. Charles E. Rosenberg, "Making It in Urban Medicine: A Career in the Age of Scientific Medicine," *Bulletin of the History of Medicine* 64 (1990): 171. Paul Starr cites several surveys that show that physician incomes at the turn of the twentieth century were not very high. See Starr, *The Social*

Transformation of American Medicine: The Rise of a Sovereign Profession and the Making of a Vast Industry (New York: Basic Books, 1982), pp. 84–85.

22. Of Anna Sampson's practice, 63.6 percent (twenty-one births of thirty-three sampled) occurred in her own town of Stoughton, a small village in southern Dane County. But like the rural midwives who delivered more than one baby, Sampson occasionally attended a birth further from home. Most of these deliveries were close to Stoughton. In addition, the majority of families who called Anna Sampson were Norwegian-born: 60.6 percent of her parturient patients had been born in Norway, and 9.1 percent were Swedish-born. However, ethnicity does not explain why Sampson might have traveled to Madison. The Madison patients that Sampson attended were neither Scandinavian nor American-born. Two patients were German-born, and one woman had been born in Ireland. Perhaps these families had lived in Stoughton and knew of Sampson's expertise prior to moving to Madison. Birth Records, Dane County, Wisconsin, Filed with Dane County Vital Records Office, City-County Building, Madison, Wisconsin (hereafter referred to as Birth Records, Dane County, DCVRO).

23. Eugene Declerq found that several midwives in Lawrence, Massachusetts, had citywide practices. See Declerq, "The Nature and Style of Practice of Immigrant Midwives in Early Twentieth-Century Massachusetts," *Journal of Social History* 19 (1985): 125.

24. U.S. Department of Commerce, Bureau of the Census, *Twelfth Census of the United States, 1900,* Manuscript Schedule, Madison, Wisconsin, (Microfilm).

25. The Jaeger family had moved to Madison by 1886, when they were listed for the first time in the City Directory (*Madison City Directory,* W. Hogg, Publishers, 1886).

26. The numbers of births attended by Dane County midwives for a total given year are not estimates; for a given sample year in Dane county, every birth was coded.

27. Caroline Jaeger, Midwife File, WSHS.

28. The Jaegers were listed in the 1919 *Madison City Directory* (Milwaukee: Wright Directory Co., 1919).

29. According to her advertisements in the city directories, Jaeger attended births in the city from 1890 through about 1915. See classified advertisements for "Midwives," *Madison City Directory,* various publishers.

30. These midwives' practices were determined from aggregating each practitioner's births by year and by ward.

31. "Active" midwives for this analysis were those midwives who delivered more than ten total babies in the sampled months for each year. Ninety-six Milwaukee midwives fit this description. The analysis was computed using only active midwives for two reasons. First, these women could be considered the most "professional" of any of the midwives, and the results of the analysis of their practice conceivably would show the broadest limits of midwifery practice. The second reason for using active midwives had to do with the limitations imposed by statistical analysis. The most valid analysis depends on having a representative number of values. A midwife with three deliveries, for example, might be recorded with a very large index, and yet the explanation for this number could be simply that she attended her own daughter across town. The locality index was a mathematical index computed by determining which ward the attendant lived in and which wards she practiced in. The index was then

computed by weighting the number of deliveries in wards relative to the midwife's own home ward. Any delivery in the midwife's own ward weighted the delivery by zero, deliveries in wards contiguous to the home ward gave a weight of one, two wards away gave a weight of two, and so forth. The weighted deliveries were then added together, and the entire sum was divided by the total number of deliveries. The resulting index then gave an approximation of the ward distance a practitioner traveled for an average delivery. Thus, a score of zero meant that the midwife never left her own ward to deliver a baby, while a score of one meant that the average distance the midwife traveled to a case was one ward away from her home. While ward boundaries are admittedly a crude measurement of neighborhoods, they provided an easily measured way to determine how far away a midwife traveled to attend her patients. Moreover, Roger D. Simon's work on Milwaukee neighborhoods, "The City-Building Process: Housing and Services in New Milwaukee Neighborhoods, 1880–1910," *Transactions of the American Philosophical Society* 68, pt. 5 (1978), also used wards to analyze the growth of neighborhoods. He showed that the clustering of ethnic and occupational groups roughly corresponded to ward divisions.

32. Graf's exact index was 1.998. Information about her comes from the 1900 census and from the midwives listed in the Milwaukee Health Department's Physician File, Milwaukee Public Library, Archives Section, Milwaukee, Wisconsin. Graf registered on August 10, 1891. The 1900 census noted that she did not speak English.

33. Mrs. Bernaski lived at 893 Sobieski; many of her births were located up and down that street. She registered with the Milwaukee City Health Department in 1887 and reported that she had trained with a physician (Physicians' Register, Milwaukee Public Library).

34. Roger Simon's work on Milwaukee neighborhoods showed distinct communities of individual ethnic groups in Milwaukee in 1905 ("The City-Building Process," pp. 20–21, maps 4, 5).

35. In 1870, 47 percent of the citizens of Milwaukee were foreign-born. Germans comprised the largest group: 32 percent of the population had been born in Germany. The British and Irish were a much smaller group, together making up 8 percent of the population (U.S. Census, *Ninth, 1870,* vol. 1, *Population,* 386–391).

36. Only the German-born Emilie Roller, who lived in a southside ward, attended more than a few Polish women.

37. Of the total number of Polish immigrants in Milwaukee County in 1900, 88.34 percent (15,588 of 17,644) were from the German parts of Poland (U.S. Census, *Twelfth, 1900,* vol. 1, *Population,* pt. 1, pp. 794–795).

38. The percentages are from the 1900 census (p. 527–528; 794–795) and the 1920 census (U.S. Census, *Fourteenth, 1920,* vol. 1, *Population,* pt. 1, p. 47).

39. The trend was even more pronounced for the four active Madison midwives. All of these midwives attended more American-born patients than women from any other ethnic group (57.5 percent of their practice). Germans made up the next largest group for each midwife: the mean for the four midwives was 28.1 percent German patients. But the differences around the mean were related to the length of time each midwife had been in practice. Maria Jessberger, who probably began her practice in Madison as early as 1865, had the largest percentage of German patients, 40 percent. On the other hand, Dora Kuehne, who did not begin to deliver babies until around 1890, had the lowest percentage of German patients, 21.3 percent.

40. The only exceptions to this close correlation were the two midwives from Austria-Hungary and the one American-born midwife. For the two midwives from Austria-Hungary, though 80 percent of their patients were from Austria-Hungary, they delivered only an average of 12 babies in a three-month period. The American-born midwife, Hattie Karsten, was an interesting anomaly that nonetheless proves my point about neighborhood practice. A second-generation German, she lived in Milwaukee's third ward from at least 1895 through 1920. A graduate of the Milwaukee School of Midwifery in 1895, she registered two times with the city health department (January 14, 1895, and September 28, 1907). Despite her training and registration efforts, however, she maintained a relatively small, neighborhood-based practice in the years that she was traced. Her 1900 practice was small—she attended four women in a three-month period, two American-born and two from Europe. By 1920, the third ward was largely populated by Italian immigrants. These women, however, used midwives extensively, and despite what must have been a substantial language barrier, they called on Hattie Karsten. In 1920, she attended twelve patients in a three-month period, all but one Italian-born. However, Mrs. Karsten was one of the only midwives to be employed extensively by an ethnic group to which she did not belong. Furthermore, these patients came from her own ward. Thus like all Milwaukee midwives, her practice had remained in her own neighborhood. (See Physicians' Register, Milwaukee Public Library; Birth Records, Milwaukee County, 1895, 1900, 1905, 1910, 1915, 1920.)

41. Use of cohort analysis helps to explain the decrease in period measures of the number of midwife-attended births between 1870 and 1920. A period measure analyzes data during a specified brief period of time, usually one year. Period data (which actually is cross-sectional data involving many cohorts) provide a current annual "picture" with respect to the event or characteristic under consideration. A cohort, on the other hand, consists of a group of individuals who experienced the same significant demographic event during a specified period of time, and who may be identified as a group at successive later dates on the basis of this common demographic experience. In contrast to period data, cohort data provide a lifetime picture for a cohort or a time series of cohorts with respect to the relevant variable. For a lengthy, technical, but careful description of both of these important demographic techniques, see Henry S. Shryock, Jacob S. Siegel, et al. (Edward G. Stockwell, ed.) *The Methods and Materials of Demography,* condensed ed. (New York: Academic Press, 1976), pp. 550–553.

42. Of the less-active urban midwives, 167 were traced to the census study on midwives. A chi-square analysis of each group of midwives by birthplace revealed no significant differences ($X^2 = 8.06$, 9 df, significance $= 0.5278$). T-tests revealed no differences between the groups in either the numbers of the ages of oldest or youngest children. (The mean number of children in the active group was 2.7; for the less active group, the mean was 2.9. For the active group, the mean age of the oldest child was 17.4 and the mean age of the youngest was 9.0; the eldest children of the less active midwives were an average 16.0 years and the youngest were an average 8.7 years old.)

43. There was no difference in the ethnic backgrounds of each group. A chi-square analysis of midwives' birthplace by the categorical variable less than 40 sampled births/more than 40 sampled births was not significant (chi-square $= 8.06$; significance $= 0.528$). The mean number of sampled deliveries for the less active German

midwives was 12.85; the mean for the Polish group was 14.57. This was not significantly different (*t*-value = − 0.73, 2-tail probability = 0.47).

44. In my sample, 173 midwives who attended less than forty total births also registered with the Milwaukee Health Department.

45. The Milwaukee Health Department's Physicians' Register provided information on country of training. Using a file consisting of midwives who appeared in both the Health Department Registration file and the Births file, I created three groups: trained in Milwaukee, trained in the United States (not Milwaukee), and trained in Europe. A one-way analysis of variance showed significant differences among these groups in the mean numbers of births attended. Midwives trained in Milwaukee oversaw a mean 27.25 births, those trained elsewhere in the United States attended a mean of 39.79 births, and those trained in Europe attended an average of 47.75 (significant at 0.002 level, with an *f*-ratio of 6.38). A Scheffe procedure showed that the foreign-trained midwives' mean was significantly different from the Milwaukee-trained midwives' mean.

46. For midwives who could be located in both the census and the birth records, the average number of deliveries for the more active group was 76.60, while the mean for the less active group was 12.98. A *t*-test of means was highly significant: *t*-value = 14.73, 2-tail probability = 0.0001. Within each group, the size of a midwife's practice could be predicted by the midwife's age. Thus, for German midwives, a *t*-test of age by the size of practice was highly significant (mean age of more active group = 49.4, mean age of less active group = 40.83, *t*-value = 3.29, 2-tail probability = 0.002). For the Polish midwives, the same effect could be found (mean age of more active group = 49.40, mean age of less active group = 40.82; *t*-value = 3.29, 2-tail probability = 0.002). There were no significant differences in mean ages, however, among the different ethnic groups within each activity group. Thus, within the less active midwives, the mean age of the German midwives was 42.50 and the mean age of the Polish midwives was 40.83, which was not significantly different (*t*-value = 0.82, 2-tail probability = 0.415).

47. A chi-square analysis of midwives' birthplace by the size of their practice (made into a categorical variable of less than forty births and more than forty births) found no significant differences among the ethnic backgrounds of the midwives (chi-square = 8.06, significance = 0.528). But an analysis of the midwife's appearance in the census did show significant differences. When each group was cross-tabulated by census year, a chi-square test showed significant differences (X^2 = 23.95 with 4 *df*, significance = 0.0001). The differences could be explained by examining the expected versus the actual frequencies in each cell: in the less active group in 1905, 6.9 women were expected, but the actual count was 10; and in 1910, the expected frequency was 34 and the actual number equaled 40. In 1880, however, 29.1 midwives from this group would have been expected, but the actual number was only 18. This same age-related effect was shown in an overall test of midwives' ages. The mean age of the more active group when identified in the census was 47.07, the mean age of the less active group was 41.89. A *t*-test of means showed significant differences between these two groups (*t* = 3.89, 239 *df*, 2-tail probability = 0.0001). The groups tested were those Milwaukee midwives who could be found in both the census and the birth records (total *n* = 241).

48. A *t*-test of means was significant: *t* = − 4.94, 243 *df*, probability = 0.0001.

49. A one-way analysis of variance showed significant differences among the groups

at the 0.0009 level, with an *f*-ratio of 7.2663. (The mean graduation date for midwives trained elsewhere in the United States was 1886. A Scheffe procedure for a multiple range test showed significant differences between the foreign-trained group and both the Milwaukee and the other-U.S. group.)

50. Using those midwives who could be identified in both the census and the birth records, the mean percentage of German patients for the active group of German midwives was 61.8 percent, while the mean percentage of American patients was 27.7 percent. For the less active group of German midwives, the mean percentage of German patients was 50.4 percent, and the mean percentage of American patients was 36.1. In a *t*-test of means, these figures were significantly different. For the mean percentages of German patients, the *t*-value = 2.61, with a 2-tail probability = 0.010; (*f*-value = 2.54). For the mean percentages of American patients, the *t*-value was −2.28, with a 2-tail probability of 0.024. In both cases, the separate variance estimate was used.

51. Though the actual percentages of German-born and Polish-born patients dropped for the less active group relative to the more active group, no statistical significance could be shown. For the Polish midwives with German patients, the mean for the more active group was 35.6 percent, versus a mean of 27.1 percent for the less active group. Yet a *t*-test of means was not significant (*t*-value = 0.82, with 2-tail probability = 0.418). For the Polish midwives with Polish patients, the results were similar: the mean for the more active group was 40.0; for the less active group, the mean was 33.7; (*t*-value = 0.53, with 2-tail probability = 0.599—not significant). A test of changes for the percentage of American patients showed little change: the mean for the more active group was 11.9; for the less active group the mean was 12.3 (*t*-value = −0.10, 2-tail probability = 0.925).

52. Judy Barrett Litoff's pioneering study of American midwives emphasizes the physician debates at the turn of the twentieth century. She stresses the cultural and language differences among midwives that helped keep them from forming groups on their own behalf. Midwives, she argues, were reliant upon others to organize them or to write articles about midwife affairs. At the same time, physician opponents to midwives were better organized and more articulate. See Litoff, *American Midwives, 1860 to the Present* (Westport, Conn.: Greenwood Press, 1978), pp. 106–107, 113.

53. Eugene Declerq did examine some of the demographic facets of midwifery practice. However, he focused on only one small northeastern city, and because of problems in gathering data, he followed a limited number of practitioners for a short time. His study began in 1896 and ended in 1914, when all the midwives in the city were prosecuted under the terms of an 1894 Massachusetts state law that forbade anybody but physicians from attending a childbirth. Like my study of Wisconsin midwives, Declerq concluded that midwifery practice in Lawrence, Massachusetts, was centered in the immigrant community, particularly among the Italians, and that it was mostly a neighborhood matter (Declerq, "The Nature and Style of Practice of Immigrant Midwives," pp. 113–129).

54. Judith Walzer Leavitt, *Brought to Bed: Childbearing in America, 1750–1950* (New York: Oxford University Press, 1986); see also Sylvia D. Hoffert, *Private Matters: American Attitudes toward Childbearing and Infant Nurture in the Urban North, 1800–1860* (Urbana: University of Illinois Press, 1989).

55. See, for example, Chapin, "The Control of Midwifery," pp. 156–158; Duke, *Infant Mortality,* p. 32; Davis, *Immigrant Health,* p. 240.

5. Educating Physicians

1. H. Reineking, "President's Address," *Transactions of the State Medical Society of Wisconsin* 33 (1899): 66.

2. Ibid., p. 67.

3. Rudolph W. Holmes, "Midwife Practice—An Anachronism," *Illinois Medical Journal* 37 (1920): 29, 30. Frances E. Kobrin attributes the significant decline of midwifery to the success of physicians like Dr. Holmes, who wanted to elevate obstetrics to a medical specialty. Kobrin, "The American Midwife Controversy: A Crisis of Professionalization," *Bulletin of the History of Medicine* 40 (1966): 350–363.

4. C. A. Harper, *Twentieth Report of the State Board of Health of Wisconsin (1903–1904)* (Madison: State Printing Office, 1905), p. 143, table 11. These percentages are based on the returns for the nine months from January 1, 1904, through September 30, 1904, shown as raw numbers in Table 11. This was the first State Board of Health Report to give statewide totals on the number of midwife and physician-assisted births.

5. Dorothy Reed Mendenhall, "Prenatal and Natal Conditions in Wisconsin," *Wisconsin Medical Journal* 15 (1917): 357. The specific figures are 12.9 percent for the entire state and 25.7 percent for city births.

6. Judy Barrett Litoff, *American Midwives, 1860 to the Present,* Contributions in Medical History no. 1 (Westport, Conn.: Greenwood Press, 1978), pp. 136, 139.

7. Paul Starr coined the term "legitimate complexity." See his *Social Transformation of American Medicine: The Rise of a Sovereign Profession and the Making of a Vast Industry* (New York: Basic Books, 1982), p. 141.

8. Physicians who delivered babies made up from 25 percent to as high as 60 percent of all physicians in practice. The percentage of doctors delivering babies grew in the last years of the nineteenth century, but varied by rural or urban location of practice. I compared the number of physicians from each year of my sample with the number of physicians listed as practicing in each county in Polk's *Medical Register and Directory of the United States and Canada* (Detroit: R. L. Polk) for the years 1886, 1890, 1896, 1900, 1906, and 1910. For the years 1916 and 1921, I obtained the numbers of practitioners in each county from the American Medical Association, *American Medical Directory* (Chicago: American Medical Association, 1916, 1921).

9. Louis Frederick Frank, *The Medical History of Milwaukee, 1834–1914* (Milwaukee: Germania Publishing Co., 1915). The "Directory of Milwaukee Physicians, 1834–1914" is found on pages 238–271. The directory provided information on physicians' schools, dates of graduation, years practiced in Milwaukee, and sometimes school of practice and specialty. This source must be used with caution, however, as some of the information on medical schools and dates attended is not accurate when compared with information provided by the physicians themselves on the state license applications. Though the license forms changed frequently to meet the new requirements of the Board, the following variables were collected from the license applications on each of the doctors: medical school attended and the year graduated; number of years of medical lectures; whether the physician had a preceptor; total number of years of medical education; number of months of hospital work (undergraduate or postgraduate); school of practice (i.e., regular, homeopathic, or eclectic); whether the physician had graduated from college; and where he or she was born. Some of the

physicians in the sample who registered after 1906 listed the number of obstetrics cases attended "under proper supervision." See Board of Medical Examiners, Physician Licenses, Series 1606, and Register of Physicians, Series 1621, Archives Division, Wisconsin State Historical Society, Madison, Wisconsin (hereafter Physician Licenses and Register of Physicians, WSHS).

10. The data included each physician's age, county and city of residence, birthplace, marital status, literacy, the numbers and ages of children present in the household, the household structure (i.e., whether relatives or boarders lived with the physician's nuclear families), and the financial status of the house where the doctor resided. The physician families were found in either the 1870, the 1880, the 1900, or the 1910 federal manuscript census schedules or in the 1905 Wisconsin state manuscript census. The linkage of 52.04 percent of the total number of physicians identified was about ten percent higher that the percentage of midwives linked to the censuses (43.4 percent).

11. See Kenneth M. Ludmerer, *Learning to Heal: The Development of American Medical Education* (New York: Basic Books, 1985), pp. 113–116; Starr, *Social Transformation of American Medicine,* p. 117.

12. Reineking, "President's Address," 66–67.

13. Regina Markell Morantz and Sue Zschoche, "Professionalism, Feminism, and Gender Roles: A Comparative Study of Nineteenth-Century Medical Therapeutics," *Journal of American History* 67 (1980): 568–588. Morantz and Zschoche compare obstetrical procedures carried out by male and female physicians.

14. Usually, but not always, the two terms were taken in each of two years. Some medical schools, however, tried to speed up the process of graduation by offering the two terms within the same year. With the increase in the length of terms to six months late in the nineteenth century, it became much harder to complete the program in one year. The practice was outlawed in Wisconsin in 1897, with passage of the Physician Registration Act, which decreed that registrants must have taken three courses of six months each, with no two courses taken within a twelve month period. Because most Wisconsin physicians attended schools where the terms were given in separate years, and because of the confusion on the licenses between terms and years, I coded the number of terms as the number of years of education.

15. The ten included the Chicago Medical School (later Northwestern University Medical School), which instituted a three-year graded program in 1868. The Chicago Medical School was one of the more popular schools among Wisconsin physicians. Throughout the 1870s, however, the three-year program at the Chicago Medical School was optional, as at other schools offering the same program, and many students still took the two-year course. See William G. Rothstein, *American Medical Schools and the Practice of Medicine: A History* (New York: Oxford University Press, 1987), pp. 103–105. For an extended discussion of medical schools in America at mid-century, see also Ludmerer, *Learning to Heal,* Chapter 1, "American Medical Education in the Mid-Nineteenth Century," pp. 9–28; and Starr, *Social Transformation of American Medicine,* pp. 112–116.

16. Ludmerer, *Learning to Heal,* pp. 47–56.

17. Starr, *Social Transformation of American Medicine,* p. 115.

18. Ludmerer, *Learning to Heal,* pp. 57–60. William Osler, whom Ludmerer and others have called the greatest American clinical teacher of all time, developed the bedside clerkship at Hopkins. Osler drew from his knowledge of the English system

of clinical clerks and surgical dressers and combined this with the German residency system for graduate physicians and the use of hospital laboratories for teaching and diagnostic purposes (ibid., pp. 60–61).

19. For 136 doctors in the pre-1905 group (22.2 percent of the total 604), no information was available about preceptorships. Preceptorships for the pre-1905 registrants pushed the total number of years of medical study to over four (mean of 4.16 years) even though the mean number of years of medical lectures was 3.54 (standard deviation equaled 1.06). The distribution of number of years of medical lectures for the pre-1905 group clustered around three years and four years.

20. Ludmerer points out that getting an undergraduate M.D. in Germany was "widely frowned upon in the United States . . . the vast majority of Americans who went to Germany . . . [sought] instead to obtain postgraduate instruction" (*Learning to Heal,* p. 33). German immigrant physicians, however, were an important group within the physician community earlier in the nineteenth century. Kathleen Neils Conzen suggests that in 1860, as many as eighteen of the city's fifty doctors had trained in Germany. See Conzen, *Immigrant Milwaukee, 1836–1860: Accommodation and Community in a Frontier City* (Cambridge: Harvard University Press, 1976), p. 122.

21. Like the regular physicians, most of the sectarians were born in this country; twenty of the thirty homeopathic doctors, for example, were native-born. A chi-square analysis showed no significant differences of school of practice by birthplace (X^2 = 6.74, 6 *df,* significance = 0.346).

22. Of these four, two declared themselves osteopaths, one described himself as both a "regular" and a "sectarian," and one physician was trained at a physiomedical school. Most of the sectarian practitioners lived in the urban areas of Wisconsin. Though one self-educated homeopathic physician practiced in Trempealeau County in the 1870s, there were no licensed homeopathic physicians in either of the rural counties of Trempealeau or Price. A chi-square analysis of school of practice by county was not significant (X^2 = 21.46, *df* = 18, significance = 0.257). To further explain this result, I examined the expected distribution of physicians versus the actual numbers. When the expected numbers of allopathic and nonallopathic physicians in each county were analyzed, the two rural counties each had only one homeopathic doctor expected. Despite the patterns of residence, however, there were very few differences between the sectarian and the regular physicians. The sectarian physicians were not significantly older than their regular counterparts: there was no significant difference in the year of graduation from medical school among all of the groups (X^2 = 28.714, *df* = 24, significance = 0.2311). For an extended discussion of sectarian medicine in nineteenth-century America, see Starr, *Social Transformation of American Medicine,* pp. 93–109.

23. Of the 604 physicians in this early group, 554 were doctors who registered with the state through the year 1905, and 50 were doctors who ended their practice in Milwaukee before 1894 and thus were found by listings in Frank, "Directory of Milwaukee Physicians." However, because Frank listed only the medical school attended, the year graduated, and the years of practice in Milwaukee, I based much of the detailed analysis in this section on the 554 licenses.

24. The chi-square analysis was significant: X^2 = 101.33, 42 *df,* significance = 0.00001.

25. There were data about specific medical school attended for 548 of the 604 physicians in the pre-1905 group (50 more physicians were known to have graduated

from some medical school that was not specified; for six physicians, the medical school was unknown). Thus, 70.3 percent of the known group attended ten medical schools.

26. In analyzing a group where information was known both from the licenses and from the census (total $n = 508$) I found that 233 of the pre-1905 group had been born in Wisconsin. This was over half of the pre-1905 physicians in this data set (408), but about 38.6 percent of the total 604 physicians identified as pre-1905 through the licenses.

27. Ernest E. Irons, *The Story of Rush Medical College* (Chicago: Board of Trustees of Rush Medical College, 1953), pp. 30–31. Rush lagged behind its chief rival, Northwestern Medical School (earlier known as Chicago Medical School), in reforming its medical curriculum. The Chicago Medical School opened its doors in 1859 with a two-year, graded curriculum. It adopted a three-year program in 1861, and in 1868, a six-month term, three-year program became mandatory. Affiliating with Northwestern University in 1869, the renamed Northwestern University Medical School adopted a seven-month term, four-year program in 1889, which became mandatory in 1892. See Leslie B. Arey, *Northwestern University Medical School, 1859–1959: A Pioneer in Educational Reform* (Evanston, Ill.: Northwestern University Medical School, 1959), p. 87. Northwestern was much less popular among Wisconsin doctors than Rush—only thirty-six doctors (6 percent) in my sample had graduated from Northwestern.

28. There are only very short histories of the Wisconsin College of Physicians and Surgeons and the Milwaukee Medical College. See Frank, *Medical History of Milwaukee,* "Medical Colleges," pp. 218–219; Ronald L. Numbers, "A Note on Medical Education in Wisconsin," in Ronald L. Numbers and Judith Walzer Leavitt, eds., *Wisconsin Medicine: Historical Perspectives* (Madison: University of Wisconsin Press, 1981), pp. 177–184. For an account of the charges brought against the Milwaukee Medical College, see Paul Cushman, Jr., "Modernizing Medical Education in Milwaukee in 1914: Contributions of a Sensational Scandal, the Flexner Report, and Student Uprising," *Bulletin of the New York Academy of Medicine* 61 (1985): 813–820. All of these histories focus on the later difficulties of these two schools and their eventual merger with Marquette University. To judge when each school moved to a four-year program, I used the evidence from the physician licenses. No records or histories of these schools describe the curriculum that was in place when the schools opened. Given the prevailing attitudes of most medical educators, both schools most likely began with a three-year, graded curriculum. The physician licenses from graduates of both schools show that graduates after 1900 attended a four-year curriculum.

29. Judith Walzer Leavitt has argued that birthing women believed that physicians offered them "scientific" practices that might save the life of both mother and baby. See Leavitt, *Brought to Bed: Childbearing in America, 1750–1950* (New York: Oxford University Press, 1986), esp. Chapter 2, "Science Enters the Birthing Room: The Impact of Physician Obstetrics," pp. 36–63.

30. George J. Engelmann, "History of Obstetrics," in B. C. Hirst, ed., *A System of Obstetrics,* 2 vols. (Philadelphia: Lea Brothers, 1888), vol. 1, p. 65; quoted by Lawrence Longo, "Obstetrics and Gynecology," in Ronald C. Numbers, ed., *Education of American Physicians: Historical Essays* (Berkeley: University of California Press, 1980), p. 216.

31. Though Harvard, Johns Hopkins, Pennsylvania, and Michigan established new standards for medical education during the 1890s and the first decade of the twentieth

century, not one of these path-breaking schools offered significant improvements in obstetric education. Even at these schools, full-time status for clinical professors of obstetrics lagged behind other education reforms. Indeed, it was not until 1919 that J. Whitridge Williams became the first full-time professor of obstetrics at Johns Hopkins. (Longo, "Obstetrics and Gynecology," pp. 205–225).

32. Horace W. Davenport, *Fifty Years of Medicine at the University of Michigan, 1891–1941* (Ann Arbor: University of Michigan Medical School, 1986), p. 372.

33. John Whitridge Williams, "Teaching Obstetrics," *Bulletin of the American Academy of Medicine* 3 (1897–98): 411; quoted by Lawrence D. Longo, "John Whitridge Williams and Academic Obstetrics in America," *Transactions and Studies of the College of Physicians of Philadelphia* 5 (1981): 227.

34. Eliza H. Root, "The Study and Teaching of Obstetrics," *Journal of the American Medical Association* 33 (1899): 511. Root used the pronoun "he" despite the fact that she taught female students at the Woman's Medical College of Northwestern University.

35. Ibid.

36. Ibid.

37. Ibid., p. 512.

38. Rosenberg notes that medical apprentices rarely learned from their preceptor's private obstetrical practice. Thus, most obstetrical instruction in the nineteenth century was dependent upon hospital and dispensary students. Charles E. Rosenberg, *The Care of Strangers: The Rise of America's Hospital System* (New York: Basic Books, 1987), p. 170.

39. Of the 604 physicians in this group, there were 475 physicians for whom hospital training could be determined. The mean number of months of hospital training was 7.34, with a standard deviation of 14.67. Months of hospital training seemed grouped around six-month intervals: while a few doctors reported other numbers of months of hospital experience, peaks occurred around six, twelve, eighteen, and twenty-four months of training. Physicians reporting more than twelve months of hospital training probably received most of their hospital experience as postgraduate hospital interns.

40. A one-way ANOVA showed no significant differences in the mean number of months of hospital training by county. [f-ratio = 0.4160, f-probability = 0.7416). No one county had significant numbers of physicians with no hospital training.

41. Ludmerer, *Learning to Heal,* pp. 16–18. Between 1870 and 1914, about 15,000 American doctors went to Germany for advanced medical training, particularly clinical training. Many of these physicians came from wealthy, east-coast families and came back from Europe to assume eminent positions in the medical hierarchies of their communities; others were the children of German immigrants. See Thomas Bonner, *American Doctors and German Universities* (Lincoln: University of Nebraska Press, 1963), pp. 23–24; also Ludmerer, *Learning to Heal,* p. 33.

42. Davenport, *Fifty Years of Medicine,* pp. 377–378.

43. J. C. Edgar, a prominent New York City obstetrician, developed a plan to teach obstetrics that included home deliveries. He stressed that students should learn obstetrical technique first under the direction of an instructor, but that later the student could "be assigned to the care of women at their own homes." J. C. Edgar, "The Best Method to Teach Obstetrics," *Journal of the American Medical Association* 26 (1896): 1120. By 1914, however, it appears that many schools required that a physician

accompany the student at all times. See Joseph B. DeLee, "Report of Sub-Committee for Illinois," *Transactions of the American Association for the Study and Prevention of Infant Mortality* (1914): 229.

44. Abraham Flexner considered medical student attendance at home deliveries to be a poor substitute for clinical obstetrical experience in a hospital. See Flexner, *Medical Education in the United States and Canada,* report to the Carnegie Foundation for the Advancement of Teaching (Carnegie Foundation for the Advancement of Teaching, 1910; reprint, Washington, D.C.: Science and Health Publications, 1960), p. 117.

45. Leslie B. Arey, *Northwestern University Medical School: A Pioneer in Educational Reform* (Evanston, Ill.: Northwestern University Medical School, 1959), p. 87. The school did not have regularly scheduled amphitheater clinics in obstetrics, so students were forced to find other means to obtain experience. Judith Walzer Leavitt notes that after the middle of the nineteenth century, some medical schools began to teach obstetrics by "demonstrative midwifery," in which students observed women in labor. Many schools, however, did not adopt this innovation and continued to teach obstetrics from textbooks and manikins (Leavitt, *Brought to Bed,* p. 63). For a history of the controversy surrounding the introduction of demonstrative midwifery in American medical schools, see Virginia G. Drachman, "The Loomis Trial: Social Mores and Obstetrics in the Mid-Nineteenth Century," in Judith Walzer Leavitt, ed., *Women and Health in America: Historical Readings* (Madison: University of Wisconsin Press, 1984), pp. 166–174.

46. Flexner, *Medical Education,* pp. 318–319. The Milwaukee Medical College was affiliated with Trinity Hospital, which had 75 beds when Flexner visited it in 1910. He reported that most of the patients were paying patients, which probably meant that they were off-limits to students. By 1913, Trinity Hospital had expanded to 100 beds, but of the 2,000 patients treated that year, only 56 were obstetrical cases. (Frank, *Medical History of Milwaukee,* p. 162). The Wisconsin College of Physicians and Surgeons was affiliated with St. Mary's Hospital, a Catholic institution. In 1912, the hospital treated 1,406 cases (ibid., p. 147).

47. For the Milwaukee Medical College, the pre-1905 mean was 1.94 months, with a standard deviation of 6.79. For the Wisconsin College of Physicians and Surgeons, the mean was 3.103 months, with a standard deviation of 10.0. The large standard deviations are the result of the high number of graduates who reported no hospital time at all.

48. Flexner, *Medical Education,* pp. 318–319.

49. Leavitt, in her discussion of the impact of physician obstetrics, cites several cases where young physicians had never attended a live birth before they began their practice (Leavitt, *Brought to Bed,* p. 63).

50. See Ludmerer, *Learning to Heal,* pp. 72–91. Robert P. Hudson writes that "Flexner's contribution was not so much revolutionary as catalytic to an already evolving process." See Hudson, "Abraham Flexner in Perspective: American Medical Education, 1865–1910," *Bulletin of the History of Medicine* 46 (1972): 545.

51. Preceptorship status was unknown for ten cases.

52. Of the 308 physicians in the post-1905 group, 270 reported a total of four years of medical study; the mean for the entire group was 4.036, with a standard deviation of 0.605. Thus, unlike the earlier group, these physicians received all of their education at medical school.

53. A *t*-test of means showed significant differences between the earlier and the later group of sectarians: the *t*-value was −2.44, 52 *df*, with 2-tail probability of 0.018.

54. A *t*-test of means showed that there were significant differences in the number of medical lectures between the post-1905 regulars and the post-1905 sectarians (*t*-value = −2.04, 320 *df*, 2-tail probability = 0.042.

55. Ludmerer notes that homeopathy began to lose popularity in the 1890s, "and within twenty years it vanished as a significant competitor to 'regular' medicine" (*Learning to Heal*, p. 94). Other less prominent medical sects "were also rapidly falling into eclipse" in the 1890s (pp. 94–95). See also Martin Kaufman, *Homeopathy in America: The Rise and Fall of a Medical Heresy* (Baltimore: Johns Hopkins University Press, 1971). Paul Starr argues, however, that the turn of the twentieth century marked both a point of acceptance of sectarian medicine as well as its moment of incipient disintegration. There were twenty-two homeopathic medical schools in 1900, but by 1918, the number had fallen to six. The number of students enrolled in eclectic medical schools peaked in 1904 at 1,000; by 1913, it had fallen to 256 (*Social Transformation of American Medicine*, p. 107). Starr attributes this decline to the growth of science, which "reinforced the effect of new institutional relations, laying the ground for a new professional consensus" (p. 102).

56. The Milwaukee Medical College began its reforms in 1907, when the school became part of Marquette University. However, this affiliation was only nominal—the University had very little direct control over its new departments of medicine and dentistry, and the forty professors of the medical school, by holding the school's $150,000 of capital stock, effectively dictated policy. To upgrade the Wisconsin College of Physicians and Surgeons and to provide money for the school's curriculum and physical plant, the school's stockholders in 1906 surrendered their stock to the college's trustees. Frank, *Medical History of Milwaukee*, pp. 218–221.

57. Flexner, *Medical Education*, pp. 318–319.

58. Frank, *Medical History of Milwaukee*, pp. 223–224.

59. For a short description of the problems with medical education in Milwaukee, see Cushman, "Modernizing Medical Education in Milwaukee in 1914," 813–820; Frank provides a somewhat longer description of the history of each school in his *Medical History of Milwaukee*, pp. 218–227. By 1920, Marquette University Medical School's Dean, Dr. Louis J. Jermain, had built up the school to the point where he had managed to raise an endowment of one million dollars. However, a bitter quarrel in the early 1920s between the university's Jesuit priests and the medical school's staff over the question of therapeutic abortions led to the mass resignation of many of the medical school's professors. By 1926, when he resigned as Dean, Jermain had again rebuilt the faculty to respectability. See Numbers, "A Note on Medical Education in Wisconsin," pp. 182–183.

60. Arey, *Northwestern University Medical School*, pp. 191–194; Bonner, *Medicine in Chicago*, p. 117.

61. The *t*-test of means for Rush was significant: *t*-value = −2.37, 132 *df*, 2-tail probability = 0.019. Northwestern proved difficult to analyze in a similar manner. A cross-tabulation of months in the hospital by graduation date showed that prior to 1906, few students spent any time in the hospital. Although some early graduates did report hospital experience, it was in discrete six-, twelve-, or eighteen-month intervals, leading to the conclusion that this was probably postgraduate hospital time. After 1906, most students reported having between one and twelve months of hospital

time, and a few had between a year and two years. With the postgraduate experience of the early group skewing the mean for the entire group, a simple *t*-test for months of hospital time by Northwestern students showed no change between the pre- and post-1905 groups.

62. Arey, *Northwestern University Medical School,* pp. 193–194.

63. Flexner, *Medical Education,* p. 117.

64. Ibid., p. 118.

65. Williams sent surveys to 120 schools; 43 responded.

66. Of the 43 schools that responded, 15 required at least one year of college; 16 required a high-school diploma; 11 replies came from schools deemed "not acceptable" by the Council on Medical Education of the American Medical Association; and one was from a Canadian medical school.

67. J. Whitridge Williams, "Medical Education and the Midwife Problem in the United States," *Journal of the American Medical Association* 58 (1912): 1–7.

68. Ibid., p. 1.

69. Ibid., p. 3.

70. Ibid., p. 5.

71. Ibid., p. 7. Williams also declared that the public needed education about the dangers of poorly trained doctors so that they would begin to demand only competent obstetricians. Furthermore, charitable and semicharitable hospital facilities he said should be increased to accommodate the needs of both poor women and those of moderate means. By a "real professor," Williams undoubtedly meant a full-time clinical professor. But even at Johns Hopkins, only a few clinical departments had full-time clinical professors; a plan to implement full-time clinical faculty met with bitter opposition from many of the clinical faculty when it was proposed in 1913. Williams later occupied the first clinical chair of obstetrics at Hopkins in 1919. See discussion of the full-time plan in Rothstein, *American Medical Schools,* pp. 162–168.

72. Longo, "John Whitridge Williams and Academic Obstetrics," p. 221. Longo gives most of the credit for this change to J. Whitridge Williams because Williams trained a large number of academic obstetricians, wrote *Obstetrics,* the leading textbook in the field, and made many scientific contributions in the field of obstetric pathophysiology.

73. See, for example, D. N. Danforth, "Contemporary titans: Joseph Bolivar DeLee and John Whitridge Williams," *American Journal of Obstetrics and Gynecology* 120 (1974): 577–588. Like Longo, Danforth seems to give more credit to Williams in terms of his contributions to teaching obstetrics. Morris Fishbein's biography of DeLee, *Joseph Bolivar DeLee: Crusading Obstetrician,* with Sol Theron DeLee (New York, E. P. Dutton, 1949), argues that though DeLee trained "a multitude" of doctors, his students devoted themselves to the practice of clinical obstetrics, rather than taking up academic posts throughout the country (p. 21). Judith Walzer Leavitt offers a new interpretation of DeLee's contributions to American obstetrics in her "Joseph B. DeLee and the Practice of Preventive Obstetrics," *American Journal of Public Health* 78 (1988): 1353–1360.

74. The correlation coefficient was significant (0.5639, significant at 0.001) between the number of months spent in the hospital and the number of obstetrical cases attended. However, Northwestern University medical students also trained at Joseph B. DeLee's Maxwell Street Dispensary, where they participated in doing home deliveries (Arey, *Northwestern University Medical School,* pp. 203–204).

75. Four Wisconsin physicians who registered after 1905 in my sample graduated from the University of Michigan.

76. The University of Michigan Medical School had been warned in the 1920s by the Association of American Medical Colleges that it was not meeting its accreditation requirements in obstetrics (Davenport, *Fifty Years of Medicine,* p. 379). However, Davenport's description of this incident does not indicate whether or not the State Board of Registration took any action in the 1930s to force the University to improve its obstetrical teaching.

77. In the 1940s, funding difficulties kept the number of poor patients at a low level, and high fees for middle-class women kept many of them from the University of Michigan Hospital (ibid., pp. 387–388).

78. The mean number of cases for each period was greatly affected by the few instances of physicians who had attended large numbers of obstetrical cases. (The mean for 1910–1919 was 20.64, and the standard deviation was 22.63; for the period 1920–1930, the mean was 30.68, and the standard deviation was 27.31.) The median, unaffected by the large outliers, gives a reasonable estimate of the group's experience. The modal number of obstetrical cases attended is also an interesting measure for these groups: for the 1910–1919 group, six cases was the most common number reported; for the 1920–1930 group, the most common number had risen to twelve.

79. Editorial, "The Recent Trend of Puerperal Mortality," *Wisconsin Medical Journal* 25 (1926): 505–506. Though the editorial was unsigned, the writer was undoubtedly Dorothy Reed Mendenhall, as she stated in the editorial that she had investigated the question of puerperal mortality ten years before.

80. When the University of Wisconsin added third and fourth years to the medical school, they hired two clinical professors in obstetrics and gynecology, both of whom were Madison practitioners. These positions, however, were not full time; the Dean of the Medical School, Charles Bardeen, had a very inadequate budget "to attempt a bona fide full-time clinical staff." See Paul F. Clark, *The University of Wisconsin Medical School: A Chronicle, 1848–1948* (Madison: Wisconsin Medical Alumni Association and the University of Wisconsin Press, 1967), p. 38. A full-time clinical professor in surgery was chosen in 1924, but it was not until 1928, with the appointment of Dr. John Warton Harris, a protégé of J. Whitridge Williams, that the university appointed its first full-time professor in obstetrics. Despite his training at Hopkins, Harris did little research at Wisconsin, and the university continued to rely extensively on part-time clinical faculty in obstetrics (ibid., pp. 179–181).

81. I am defining medical leaders as those who were active in the Wisconsin State Medical Society and at the medical schools in the state, and who wrote of their concerns in the *Wisconsin Medical Journal.* Most of these physicians, including many of the editors of the *Journal,* were general practitioners. J. P. McMahon, the managing editor of the *Journal* in the early 1920s, however, was an active Milwaukee obstetrician.

82. Rock Sleyster, "Co-operation of State Medical Societies with the University Extension Movement," *Wisconsin Medical Journal* 14 (1915–16): 8.

83. Ibid., p. 8. Sleyster lived in Wauwatosa, a suburb of Milwaukee.

84. "Postgraduate Courses in Obstetrics," *Wisconsin Medical Journal* 20 (1922): 427–428.

85. Editorial, "Post Graduate Study," *Wisconsin Medical Journal* 25 (1926): 445–446. An editorial noted in 1922 that the Walworth County Medical Society had taken

"the full University postgraduate course in obstetrics." *Wisconsin Medical Journal* 21 (1922–23): 60. Ludmerer notes the creation of a variety of postgraduate courses that became available in the 1890s to help bring existing practitioners up to date with recent scientific advances (*Learning to Heal,* p. 94).

86. Rosemary Stevens, *American Medicine and the Public Interest* (New Haven: Yale University Press, 1971), pp. 201–203.

87. The University of Wisconsin usually had one resident in obstetrics per year up through the early 1950s (Clark, *The University of Wisconsin Medical School,* p. 182). Even as late as 1938, the University of Wisconsin program was the only approved residency in obstetrics in Wisconsin. Several Chicago hospitals offered obstetrics or obstetrics and gynecological residencies by 1938, but with a total of only sixteen places. See "Hospitals Approved for Residencies in Specialties," *Journal of the American Medical Association* 111 (1938): 838–840.

88. Stevens, *American Medicine,* p. 203.

89. Though they always supported programs for training physicians for a general practice, Wisconsin's physician leaders by the late 1920s were voicing concern about the ability of the general practitioner to absorb all of the new scientific concepts. See, for example, the editorial "The Glorified General Practitioner," *Wisconsin Medical Journal* 26 (1927): 517–518. The author of this editorial expressed sympathy for the general practitioner and the art of medicine at the same time that he noted the difficulties and the necessity of keeping up with the scientific literature in all fields.

6. Country Doctors Replace Midwives

1. W. T. Sarles, "The Country Doctor in Obstetrics," *Transactions of the State Medical Society of Wisconsin* 28 (1894): 316.

2. Ibid., p. 319.

3. Of the physicians in my study for whom a license could be found, the physician's birthplace was noted on 777. Of this 777 total, (52.4 percent) were natives of Wisconsin. Of the 598 physicians traced to the various federal and local censuses, 329 (55 percent) were born in the state. Interestingly, the percentages of Wisconsin natives traced to the censuses did not vary by urban or rural location of practice: 86 of the 156 rural doctors (55.1 percent) and 243 of the 442 urban doctors (55 percent) were natives. For the details of the physicians' licenses, see Chapter 5. For the census study, physician families were found in either the 1870, the 1880, the 1900, or the 1910 federal manuscript census schedules or in the 1905 Wisconsin state manuscript census; for the licenses, see Board of Medical Examiners, Physician Licenses (Series 1606) and Register of Physicians (Series 1621), Archives Division, Wisconsin State Historical Society, Madison, Wisconsin (hereafter Physician Licenses, WSHS).

4. See Chapter 5 for a longer explication of this decision. Early in the twentieth century, the State of Wisconsin Medical Society reorganized along the guidelines established by the American Medical Association. Ronald L. Numbers points out that after this reorganization, many specialty societies were formed. These specialty groups were devoted almost exclusively to clinical medicine, and his sources reveal that they were almost all located in Milwaukee. See Numbers, "Public Protection and Self-Interest: Medical Societies in Wisconsin," in Ronald L. Numbers and Judith Walzer Leavitt, eds., *Wisconsin Medicine: Historical Perspectives* (Madison: University of Wisconsin Press, 1981), pp. 75–104.

5. While more physicians would probably have been identified in the unsampled months, the amount of months sampled for each year (either three or four) demonstrates the low level of obstetrical cases taken by most physicians before 1900. Number of physicians was obtained from the 1896, 1890, 1896, 1900, 1906, and 1910 editions of Polk's *Medical Register and Directory of the United States and Canada* (Detroit: R.L. Polk) and the American Medical Association's *American Medical Directory* for 1916 and 1921 (Chicago: American Medical Association).

6. A *t*-test of means found that these monthly averages were significant (*t*-value = −4.97, *df* = 67.61, 2-tail probability = 0.0001). There were 62 doctors in the rural counties, 832 in Milwaukee.

7. A. H. Bill, "The New Obstetrics," *American Journal of Obstetrics and Gynecology* 23 (1932): 155; quoted by Lyle G. McNeile, "Trends in American Obstetrics during the First Third of This Century," *Journal of the American Medical Association* 107 (1936): 173.

8. Many articles in the *Transactions of the State Medical Society of Wisconsin* (later the *Wisconsin Medical Journal*) in the period from about 1890 to 1930 focused on the need to claim obstetrics as a scientifically based part of medicine. From the tone of the articles, however, it was apparent that the public, specifically birthing women in cash-strapped rural Wisconsin, were not ready to believe that the doctor ought to be employed for routine maternity cases. See, for example, the article written by Dr. J. R. L. Barnett, of Neenah, Wisconsin. He complained of "the practice of thousands of thrifty households, which grudge even the modest charge of the village auntie; and think the doctor, if not a superfluity, at least an extravagance not to be endured, unless the matter come to the point of instrumental interference, when they invoke his special skill willingly, even with eagerness." "Puerperal Hemorrhage: Its Treatment in Extremity," *Transactions of the State Medical Society of Wisconsin* 33 (1899): 80. Dr. L. G. Armstrong, in discussing Dr. Sarles's paper, noted that he had spent a considerable amount of time trying to persuade his neighbors to abandon the "old granny in the neighborhood, who happened to be present just because she was good-natured, and was pretty good at dressing the baby afterwards." He argued instead that "there is something to be done more than to sit down and trust simply to nature." Armstrong, "Discussion" to Sarles, "The Country Doctor in Obstetrics," pp. 322–323.

9. Judith Walzer Leavitt, *Brought to Bed: Childbearing in America, 1750–1950* (New York: Oxford University Press, 1986).

10. To measure the process of change from midwives to general practitioners, this chapter uses birth certificates filed by physicians who were practicing in the rural areas of this study. The data from the birth certificates provided information on both the pace of practice and the geographical extent of physicians' obstetrical work. In addition, the information on practice was linked to the physicians' licenses and to the censuses to assess the impact of medical education and physicians' ethnic backgrounds on their obstetrical practice. For a complete description of these sources, see the appendix.

11. Paul Starr, *The Social Transformation of American Medicine: The Rise of a Sovereign Profession and the Making of a Vast Industry* (New York: Basic Books, 1982), p. 141.

12. A Children's Bureau survey of maternity conditions in Marathon County, Wisconsin, revealed that many doctors had passed up routine obstetrics. The physicians told the interviewers that they did not "like that kind of work" and so they turned it over to a local midwife. Florence Brown Sherbon and Elizabeth Moore, *Maternity*

and Infant Care in Two Rural Counties in Wisconsin, U.S. Department of Labor, Children's Bureau Publication no. 46 (Washington, D.C.: Government Printing Office, 1919), pp. 32–33.

13. For example, B. F. Dodson, a Berlin, Wisconsin, physician, wrote, "No adequate fee is paid the doctor by those able to reward him for his services in this very important hour in the household. The entrance into the sick chamber of one who is to calm their fears through his known ability and success, deserves more than the small pittance usually paid the country physician." B. F. Dodson, "Some Responsibilities in the Line of Obstetrical Work," *Transactions of the State Medical Society of Wisconsin* 35 (1901): 355. Many articles on obstetrics written at the end of the nineteenth century complained of the length of time needed for obstetrical cases and the low fees that these cases engendered. Indeed, one of the primary arguments of physicians who opposed midwives was that their charges depressed physicians' fees for maternity services. Dr. Dodson, for example, felt this way. For an extended discussion of this issue, see Judy Barrett Litoff, *American Midwives, 1860 to the Present,* Contributions in Medical History, no. 1 (Westport, Conn.: Greenwood Press, 1978).

14. "George N. Hidershide, M.D.," in *History of Trempealeau County, Wisconsin,* compiled by Franklyn Curtiss-Wedge, edited by Eben Douglas Pierce (Chicago: H. C. Cooper, Jr., & Co., 1917), pp. 754–757.

15. Ibid. Details on Dr. Hidershide's obstetrical practice are from the sampled vital records of Trempealeau County. In 1915, he attended nine births in a six-month period, the most he ever oversaw.

16. The year beginning practice in Figure 6.2 represents the five-year interval up to and including the year depicted. Thus, the year 1890 on this graph represents all those doctors in my sample who began their medical practice between 1886 and 1890. The year 1875 includes all the years before 1876.

17. The date beginning practice was figured from the date of registration and the number of years of medical practice indicated on the physicians' licenses. The date beginning obstetrical practice was calculated from the date of the first delivery in my birth sample. Because I sampled every five years, I considered a physician to have delayed starting his obstetrical practice if he did not appear in my birth sample ten or more years after beginning his medical practice.

18. Physicians' Licenses, WSHS. The correspondence between these two dates was subject to the problem of determining where a physician began his practice. There would be lag time, of course, if a physician had been in practice elsewhere before he moved into my study area.

19. Indeed, I found some physicians who were not listed in the standard directories. The AMA's *American Medical Directory* for 1921 listed thirty-five doctors practicing in Trempealeau and Price Counties; there were forty doctors in my sample. The data set from Dane County was not used in this analysis because the sampled years in the Dane County data set did not correspond to those in Trempealeau and Price Counties. As detailed in the appendix, the Dane County data did not include the years 1905, 1915, and 1920. However, the Dane County data is used in this chapter in separate analyses.

20. Rosemary Stevens, *American Medicine and the Public Interest* (New Haven: Yale University Press, 1971), p. 147.

21. Twenty-eight (72 percent) of the thirty-nine doctors delivering babies in 1900 in these counties were new doctors.

22. In 1890, there were only four physicians in Price County; by 1896, there were five, including Dr. Fenelon.

23. Fourteen physicians were practicing in Price County in 1921 (*American Medical Directory*, 1921). I found twelve of them delivering babies in my sample. Information on Dr. Fenelon comes from his state medical license (Physicians' Licenses, WSHS) and from the birth certificates that he signed. He was unusual in relation to many country doctors in having attended college before going to medical school.

24. Starr, *Social Transformation of American Medicine*, pp. 69–71.

25. Paul Starr describes the economic difficulties of early nineteenth-century physicians. Many physicians in these years found it hard to support themselves solely from medical practice, so they adopted a second occupation to support themselves and their families (Starr, *Social Transformation of American Medicine*, p. 65). In the late nineteenth century, with the transportation revolution and the advent of telephones, the medical market was transformed. According to Starr, "the reduction of indirect prices from the local transportation revolution and the rise of cities put medical care within the income range of more people" (p. 71).

26. Armstrong, "Discussion," p. 322. Armstrong, who lived in Boscobel, in the southwestern part of the state, was a censor for the State Medical Society in 1893 and 1896. See "State Medical Society of Wisconsin. Officers and Members for 1890–1," *Transactions of the State Medical Society of Wisconsin* 24 (1890): n.p. also "State Medical Society of Wisconsin. Officers and Committees for 1895–96," *Transactions* 24 (1895): n.p.

27. C. M. Schuldt, "The Need of Maternity Service in Rural Districts," *Wisconsin Medical Journal* 19 (1920–21): 576.

28. M. V. De Wire, "The After Care of Obstetrical Cases in a Country Practice," *Wisconsin Medical Journal* 7 (1908–1909): 650. De Wire also noted the problems of dealing with emergencies in a home situation, where the family was "keeping up a running fire of questions" (p. 650).

29. B. J. Wadey, "Obstetrics in Rural Communities," *Wisconsin Medical Journal* 20 (1922): 285.

30. Ibid., p. 288. Wadey noted that midwives "are content to sit by their cases, letting Mother Nature do the work and reap the glory, while we physicians, with a license to do and with the necessary instruments at hand, are too eager to hasten the labor and get away." But this eagerness to get away, he asserted, was somewhat understandable, given the distances between patients (p. 288).

31. The following chart illustrates this point. The number of births are six-month totals attended by Dr. Fenelon (source: Birth Records, Price County, years indicated, WDHHS, Madison, Wisconsin).

Year	No. of births	No. of births in Phillips	No. of births not in Phillips
1895	29	29	0
1900	63	45	18
1905	4	2	2
1910	33	31	2
1915	37	22	15
1920	21	21	0

32. Though Dr. Sperry delivered, on average, about 20 patients in six months, only one or two were from outside the village. The year 1900 was the only exception: that year, of the 36 deliveries in a six-month period, 13 were from outside Phillips.

33. In the six sampled months of 1920, Dr. Francis attended 9 births in Keenan and 4 in Catawba.

34. Dr. Sperry attended 23 births in Phillips and 13 births in the villages of Fifield, Ogema, Prentice, and Worcester and in the township of Georgetown. Dr. Fenelon oversaw 45 births in Phillips and 18 births in the villages of Prentice, Fifield, and Worcester and in the township of Georgetown. Dr. Fenelon apparently rode a bicycle, and he also had a "cycle sort of vehicle," which could be used on the railroad tracks. A county history explains that this vehicle made his trips "to nearby villages and communities along the Wisconsin Central Railroad speedily accessible." Centennial Commission, *Centennial Phillips, Wisconsin* (Phillips, Wisconsin: privately published 1976), p. 172. County maps of the era show a road north from Phillips to Fifield, but no direct road south to Worcester, Prentice, or Ogema. See Wisconsin Central Railroad Company, "Map of Price County & Part of Lincoln, Oneida & Chippewa Counties. Wis.," Archives Division, Wisconsin State Historical Society, Madison, Wisconsin. Paul Starr argues that railroads had a significant impact on physicians' practices. Railroads, he finds, widened doctors' markets by expanding the territory they could cover. Doctors, in fact, were such frequent travelers on the railroads that some of them received travel passes in exchange for treating railroad workers' injuries. The railroads also brought patients in from a distance. Starr maintains that "naturally doctors wanted to be in towns along the routes to enjoy the benefits" (*Social Transformation of American Medicine*, p. 69).

35. Riding two defined circuits a day, they covered farms and towns all through the western part of the county. See Middleton Doctor's Day Historical Committee, *Doctor's Day in Middleton: Honoring Dr. Allen and Dr. Rowley* (privately printed, August 21, 1949).

36. Paul Starr discusses the advantages to physicians who bought cars early in the twentieth century (*Social Transformation of American Medicine*, p. 70). Dr. A. G. Rowley, A. A. Rowley's son, took over his father's practice in Middleton in 1902. See Jessica Rowley, "The Story of the Rowley Drug Store (Rowley Doctors)," dated 1955, typed manuscript in Rowley Family Papers, Wis Mss, 13 PB/22, Archives Division, State Historical Society of Wisconsin, Madison. The date of Dr. Rowley's purchase is noted in *Doctor's Day in Middleton*, p. 16.

37. M. L. Berger, "The Influence of the Automobile on Rural Health Care, 1900–1929," *Journal of the History of Medicine and Allied Sciences* 28 (1973): 319–335; cited by Guenter B. Risse, "From Horse and Buggy to Automobile and Telephone: Medical Practice in Wisconsin, 1848–1930," in Numbers and Leavitt, eds., *Wisconsin Medicine: Historical Perspectives*, p. 38. Risse finds that many mid and late nineteenth-century Wisconsin physicians accepted cases within a twenty to twenty-five mile radius (p. 28). However, my data indicate that few physicians traveled even this far, at least to maternity patients.

38. In the years that were sampled, Dr. A. A. Rowley attended an average of three cases a month, for a yearly total of thirty-five to forty-five births a year. "Birth Records," Dane County, Wisconsin, sampled years 1885–1900. Filed with Dane County Vital Records Office, City-County Building, Madison, Wisconsin (hereafter referred to as Birth Records, Dane County, DCVRO).

39. Dr. Antinous A. Rowley of Dane County, an 1867 graduate of Rush Medical College, joined his father in practice at the small railroad depot town of Middleton, Wisconsin, in 1868. Like many other nineteenth-century physicians, to make ends meet, the Rowleys ran a business in addition to maintaining their medical practice. Operating a drug and general supplies store located behind the local bank, they employed their apprentices as clerks while they were away on call. The Rowleys also took the unusual step of establishing an office away from their homes, using the rooms over the drugstore. These rooms were also used for some surgical operations. Five years after the death of Newman Rowley in 1880, his grandson, A. G. Rowley, closed the drugstore and moved his office to a building adjacent to his home. He continued, however, to dispense drugs in the course of his practice (Rowley, "The Story of the Rowley Drug Store"). All of the births attended by A. G. Rowley in 1910 were either in Middleton or in surrounding farm towns in the middle of the county.

40. In each year sampled, a few doctors delivered more than the mean numbers. However, these obstetrical caseloads were never very large. In 1880, for example, with a mean for 9 physicians of 7.7 births per year, 3 doctors attended 12 or more births during the year, with Dr. L. D. Clark of Stoughton attending the most, at 19. In 1890, 17 physicians delivered an average of 11.28 births, and 7 of these doctors had an average of more than 1 birth per month, but A. A. Rowley and C. K. Jayne represented the high end of 3 births per month. In 1900, with 45 doctors practicing obstetrics in the county, the average number of births dropped to 6.15 per year; only 5 doctors delivered more than 1 birth per month, and only Dr. A. A. Rowley delivered 3 babies per month. By 1910, the average was still less than 1 birth per month; 4 doctors delivered more than 3 babies per month, and Dr. B. W.Shaw attended 63 births. As Chapter 7 will show, however, even Dr. Shaw's 1910 total was only half of what an obstetrical specialist in these years would expect to attend. The low means for all of these years also reflect the fact that many rural general practitioners attended only a few births per year.

41. To study the geographic aspects of practice in rural Dane County, I divided the county into six zones, with Madison at the center. The location of each rural doctor's cases was compared with his residence. In every year studied (1880, 1890, 1900, and 1910), the cases matched up with the doctor's residence or the adjacent areas. The location of the obstetrical cases of doctors living outside of Dane County also showed this tight local pattern. Their cases were almost always in the areas just adjacent to their counties. It is also interesting that very few of these rural doctors ever delivered an obstetrical case in Madison.

42. Some physicians rode sleighs through open fields in the winter, cutting the fences surrounding these fields when necessary. Keeping warm in winter was a major concern. For a bone-chilling description, see Risse, "From Horse and Buggy," p. 28. Starr finds that the high costs of travel made rural medical practice very lonely and isolated. But by the beginning of the twentieth century, telephones, automobiles, and paved roads enabled physicians to cut down on their travel costs. Patients could also reach medical help more easily. Starr, *Social Transformation of American Medicine,* pp. 68–71.

43. Charles E. Rosenberg, "The Therapeutic Revolution: Medicine, Meaning, and Social Change in Nineteenth-Century America," in Morris J. Vogel and Charles E. Rosenberg, eds., *The Therapeutic Revolution: Essays in the Social History of American Medicine* (Philadelphia: University of Pennsylvania Press, 1979), pp. 3–25; John

Harley Warner, *The Therapeutic Perspective: Medical Practice, Knowledge, and Identity in America, 1820–1885* (Cambridge: Harvard University Press, 1986).

44. Rosenberg, "The Therapeutic Revolution," p. 11.

45. The number born in Wisconsin by far exceeded the number of physicians born anywhere else, even those born elsewhere in the United States (*n* = 28). A one-way chi-square test showed that this was highly significant (chi-square = 157.36, 6 *df*, significance = 0.0001).

46. Paul Starr and Ronald L. Numbers both point out the low status of physicians in the nineteenth century. See Starr, *Social Transformation of American Medicine,* and Numbers, "The Fall and Rise of the American Medical Profession," in Judith Walzer Leavitt and Ronald L. Numbers, eds., *Sickness and Health in America: Readings in the History of Medicine and Public Health,* 2nd ed., rev. (Madison: University of Wisconsin Press, 1985), pp. 185–196.

47. Franklyn Curtiss-Wedge, compiler, and Eben Douglas Pierce, ed., *History of Trempealeau County, Wisconsin* (Chicago: H. C. Cooper, Jr. & Co., 1917), p. 225. Briggs, described as a self-trained homeopath, was one of the four big landowners in early Arcadia (ibid, pp. 224–230). It is interesting to note that the editor of this county history, Eben Douglas Pierce, was a physician.

48. Ibid., pp. 754–757. In April 1894, Dr. Hidershide strung a telephone wire from his home to his office, thus becoming the first person in Trempealeau County to have a telephone (p. 267).

49. Ibid., pp. 253, 581–582.

50. Ibid., p. 503.

51. Ibid., p. 521.

52. The legislature voted to establish a state board of health in 1876. The board was given broad powers to supervise the "health and life of the citizens of the state." The mechanism for the enforcement of these powers lay in a system of local city and village health boards that would systematically report on illnesses and death. See Dale E. Treleven, "One Hundred Years of Health and Healing in Rural Wisconsin," in Ronald L. Numbers and Judith Walzer Leavitt, eds., *Wisconsin Medicine,* pp. 133–154; quote is from p. 138.

53. Treleven argues that late nineteenth-century rural health officers had great difficulty in enforcing quarantines and community clean-up campaigns. While this undoubtedly was the case, he also shows that physicians increased their presence in the community by serving on these boards. An 1883 law amended the 1876 one by requiring each city council and village or town board to appoint a physician to the post of health officer. By 1895, almost every locality in the state had set up a local health board (1,219 of 1,256 towns, villages, and cities) (Treleven, "Rural Wisconsin," pp. 138–139). Lee Anderson's recent study of the public health movement in late nineteenth-century Iowa traces the interrelationship between politics, middle-class morality, and the new science of public health. He argues, however, that much of this work was carried on by "medical elites" within the state, and that the "rank and file" of Iowa's doctors often refused to "be led in directions that elites wanted to go." See Anderson, " 'Headlights Upon Sanitary Medicine': Public Health and Medical Reform in Late Nineteenth-Century Iowa," *Journal of the History of Medicine and Allied Sciences* 46 (1991): 178–200.

54. Curtiss-Wedge, *History of Trempealeau County,* p. 756.

55. Ibid., p. 521.

56. Ibid., p. 396.

57. The health officer was from Hale. Wisconsin State Board of Health, *Ninth Annual Report, 1885* (Madison, 1886), pp. 130–131, 225; quoted by Treleven, "Rural Wisconsin," p. 139.

58. Drs. Jegi, Peterson, E. A. Olson, and Hidershide were among those who acted as local Trempealeau County health officers (Curtiss-Wedge, *History of Trempealeau County*, pp. 503, 581, 756).

59. Judith Walzer Leavitt has argued convincingly that nineteenth-century women, fearing the mortal effects of childbirth, opted for a physician who could bring "science into the birthing room." She acknowledges, however, that her population of women was middle-class, and her sources reveal that they were predominately native-born. See Leavitt, *Brought to Bed*, esp. Chapter 2, "Science Enters the Birthing Room: The Impact of Physician Obstetrics," pp. 36–63.

60. These six doctors' own ethnic background was checked in the manuscript census. To determine the percentage of American-born patients, each physician's percentage was weighted by the number of births he attended. U.S. Department of Commerce, Bureau of the Census, *Tenth Census of the United States, 1880*, vol. 1, *Population,* p. 535.

61. Though a few rural counties in Wisconsin had populations of German, Polish, and other immigrant groups, Norwegians were the dominant immigrant group in many areas of rural Wisconsin. In 1895, Scandinavian immigrants numbered 106,900, the second largest immigrant group in the state. See Robert C. Nesbit, *Wisconsin, A History* (Madison: University of Wisconsin Press, 1973), p. 347. In 1880, Scandinavian immigrants were the largest single immigrant group in Trempealeau and Price Counties (U.S. Census, *Tenth, 1880, Population*, p. 535), and by 1900, they were the largest group in rural Dane, Trempealeau, and Price Counties. Population figures for 1900 are as follows (source: U.S. Census, *Twelfth, 1900*, vol. 1, *Population,* pp. lvii, 794–795):

Population	Dane	Price	Trempealeau
Total	69,435	9,106	23,114
Foreign	15,490	3,325	6,206
Scandinavian	7,062	1,639	4,135

The Scandinavian population in Price County was mostly Swedish. Clearly, for the rural counties of this study, Scandinavians comprised the dominant immigrant group.

62. Curtiss-Wedge, *History of Trempealeau County*, pp. 581–582; see also Physician Licenses and Birth Certificates, Trempealeau County, WSHS.

63. There were a total of twelve immigrant Norwegian and four German-born doctors in the three rural areas of my study, most of them in Trempealeau County. A. K. Olsen had come to the United States in 1886, at age 21. He graduated from Chicago's College of Physicians and Surgeons in 1894 (Curtiss-Wedge, *History of Trempealeau County*, p. 521). Budom, according to the census, had come to the United States in 1890. He registered with the State Board of Medical Examiners in 1899. In 1900, he was age 37, living in the village of Blair (U.S. Census, *Twelfth,*

1900, Manuscript Schedule [microfilm], Trempealeau County, Wisconsin; also Physician Licenses, WSHS).

64. A *t*-test of mean percentage of Scandinavian patients for physicians in Trempealeau and Price Counties showed that immigrant doctors had a practice that averaged 33.10 percent Scandinavian patients, while American-born physicians had an average of 19.75 percent. This was significant at the 0.016 level (*t*-value = 2.48, 60.64 *df*). In Dane County, four immigrant physicians came from Germany and five from Scandinavia. For the Scandinavian-born physicians, women from their homeland comprised about 23.66 percent of their practice, a figure significantly different from the German physicians (*t*-value = −2.37, 8.59 *df*, significance = 0.043) and from the American-born doctors (*t*-value = 2.18, 104 *df*, significance = 0.032). Part of the reason for the Dane County doctors' slightly smaller percentages may lie with Dane County's earlier settlement. As early as 1838, Norwegian settlers from Illinois pushed up into Dane County, while Trempealeau County was not settled until the 1860s and 1870s (Nesbit, *Wisconsin,* pp. 138–139 passim). It is probable that many of the American-born women attended by these physicians were the daughters of Scandinavian immigrants.

65. Of the physicians with immigrant parents, those of Scandinavian background comprised the largest number (*n* = 23). The next largest group were those of English or Scottish descent (*n* = 19); only 9 doctors were of German descent (Germany or Switzerland).

66. In Dane County, the eleven doctors with Scandinavian parents had significantly higher percentages of Scandinavian patients (mean of 24.6 percent). The mean for other groups was no higher than 7.09 percent Scandinavian patients (one-way ANOVA *f*-ratio of 6.56, significant at 0.0004; a Scheffe test showed that this mean was significantly different from the mean of all other groups, at 0.05 level). In Trempealeau and Price Counties, the mean percentage of Scandinavian patients for Scandinavian doctors was 36.6 percent, while the mean percentage of Scandinavian patients for doctors of other ethnic backgrounds was no higher than 29.90 percent (for the doctors with parents from the British Isles). The Scandinavian doctors' mean was significantly different (one-way ANOVA, *f*-ratio of 4.15, significant at 0.0036).

67. Armstrong, "Discussion," on Sarles, "The Country Doctor in Obstetrics," p. 323.

68. Dorothy Reed Mendenhall, "Prenatal and Natal Conditions in Wisconsin," *Wisconsin Medical Journal* 15 (1917): 357.

69. In 1900, 36.5 percent of Price County's population was foreign-born. By 1910, the numbers began to fall, but by 1920, about 26 percent of the population was still foreign-born (U.S. Census, *Twelfth, 1900,* vol. 1, *Population,* pp. 794–795; *Thirteenth, 1910,* vol. 1, *Population,* p. 824; *Fourteenth, 1920,* vol. 1, *Population,* pp. 1370–1371). Of the seventeen doctors from Price County who were found in this study, seven were born in Wisconsin, six elsewhere in the United States, and one in Scandinavia.

70. Of the twenty midwives practicing in either Trempealeau or Price County in 1920, sixteen were from Price County (Birth Records, Trempealeau and Price Counties, January–June 1920).

71. Barbara Gutmann Rosenkrantz, "The Search for Professional Order in Nineteenth-Century American Medicine," in Leavitt and Numbers, eds., *Sickness and Health,* pp. 219–232.

72. Edward Atwater demonstrated the increasing importance of education in launching and maintaining a successful practice in Rochester, New York, in the last decades of the nineteenth century. It is significant that many of Rochester's physicians received their training in regional schools: over one-third of the physicians Atwater found practicing in late nineteenth-century Rochester had trained in three schools nearby. See Edward Atwater, "The Physicians of Rochester, N.Y., 1860–1910: A Study in Professional History, II," *Bulletin of the History of Medicine* 47 (1973): 94. Of the 777 physicians in my license data set where birthplace was known, 407 (52.4 percent) were born in Wisconsin. The percentages were similar for those physicians located in the censuses: 55.1 percent of the doctors in the census study were born in the state. A recent study of physicians in late nineteenth-century Watertown, Wisconsin, shows that the key to financial success for a physician lay with local roots. See Walter J. Vanast, "Constancy, Continuity, and Curiosity: A Reassessment of the 'Low Estate' of Nineteenth-Century American Doctors," paper given at the Sixty-Sixth Annual Meeting of the American Association of the History of Medicine, Louisville, Kentucky, May 15, 1993.

7. Specializing Obstetrics

1. Henry P. Newman, "The Specialty of Obstetrics, Present Status, Possibilities and Importance," *American Journal of Obstetrics* 80 (1919): 466. Obstetricians were "disputing the ground" with more than midwives and general practitioners. In 1911, the American Medical Association formed a section entitled "Obstetrics and Gynecology." However, only a year later, the section was renamed "Obstetrics, Gynecology, and Abdominal Surgery" due to the surgical interests of many of its members and because these surgeons were fighting with general surgeons over who should operate in the abdomen. The name of the section reverted to "Obstetrics and Gynecology" in 1938. Rosemary Stevens, *American Medicine and the Public Interest* (New Haven: Yale University Press, 1971), p. 201, n. 8.

2. Dorothy Reed Mendenhall, "Prenatal and Natal Conditions in Wisconsin," *Wisconsin Medical Journal* 15 (1917): Table 4, p. 357. Interestingly, in a 1936 address, Lyle G. McNeile, the chair of the AMA's Committee on Obstetrics, Gynecology, and Abdominal Surgery, found that five trends had contributed to the growth of obstetrics as a specialty, and that opposition to midwives was one of the least important. Lyle G. McNeile, "Trends in American Obstetrics during the First Third of This Century," *Journal of the American Medical Association* 107 (1936): 173–178.

3. Edward P. Davis, quoted by George Clark Mosher, "Maternal Morbidity and Mortality in the United States," *American Journal of Obstetrics and Gynecology* 7 (1924): 295.

4. Charles M. Ellis, "The Country Doctor," *Journal of the American Medical Association* 30 (1898): 1173.

5. J. P. McMahon, "Comments," to Walter G. Darling, "Puerperal Infection," *Wisconsin Medical Journal* 14 (1915–16): 86. Frances Kobrin's pioneering article on midwives in the United States identified this problem of professional status for academic obstetricians. She connected their vehemence at eliminating midwifery with their own need to elevate the status of obstetrics, but she did not trace the specialist

physicians' campaign against general practitioners. See Kobrin, "The American Midwife Controversy: A Crisis of Professionalization," *Bulletin of the History of Medicine* 40 (1966): 350–363.

6. In 1968, 68 percent of all births were attended by an obstetrician. This percentage rose to 81 percent by 1977. National Institutes of Health and the U.S. Public Health Service, *Cesarean Childbirth*, NIH Publication no. 82-2067 (Washington, D.C.: U.S. Department of Health and Human Services, 1981), p. 80. In 1900, 39 physicians and 9 midwives attended maternity cases in Trempealeau and Price Counties. Current statistics, shown in the table below, illustrate the flight of physicians from rural practice. Indeed, if the number of midwives in Trempealeau and Price Counties at the turn of the century were added to the number of physicians, the current number of practitioners in these two rural counties would equal the number of midwives and physicians attending maternity cases in 1895 (33 in 1895).

County	Total no. of physicians	No. of FP/GP	No. of Surg. Spec.
Milwaukee	3,159	221	492
Dane	1,817	121	210
Trempealeau	22	11	1
Price	11	6	1

Entire State:
Total no. of physicians in Wisconsin in 1993:	10,701
No. of physicians involved in total patient care:	8,984
No. of physicians FP/GP:	1,679
No. of physicians specializing in Ob-Gyn:	471

The total number of physicians identified for each county were those physicians involved in total patient care, not academic or other institutional medicine. These latter types of physicians were not included in order to maintain consistency with the historical experience of most physicians, who remained doing patient care even if they were academic physicians. Milwaukee and Dane Counties, the site of the two medical schools in Wisconsin, have most of the physicians in this latter category. "FP/GP" are those doctors who identified themselves as either family practice or general practice physicians. "Surg. spec." are those physicians who identified themselves as practicing any surgical specialty, including obstetrics and gynecology. Gene Roback, Lillian Randolph, and Bradley Seidman, *Physician Characteristics and Distribution in the U.S.,* 1993 ed. (Chicago: American Medical Association, 1993), table 9, p. 183; table 12, p. 255.

7. E. F. Fish, "The Practice of Obstetrics," *Wisconsin Medical Journal* 2 (1903–4): 547.

8. My sample shows that only 26 percent of the city's physicians attended a birth in 1885, by 1895, this fraction had risen only slightly, to 32 percent. While more physicians would probably have been identified in the unsampled months, the amount

of months sampled for each year (either three or four) demonstrates the low level of obstetrical cases taken by most physicians before 1900. Number of "all physicians" was obtained from the 1890, 1896, 1900, 1906, and 1910 editions of Polk's *Medical Register and Directory of the United States and Canada* (Detroit: R.L. Polk) and the *American Medical Directory* for 1916 and 1921 (Chicago: American Medical Association).

9. Bayview, which had been settled in 1867, lay along Lake Michigan southeast of Milwaukee. However, by 1890, the village had become Milwaukee's seventeenth ward. Bayrd Still, *Milwaukee: The History of a City* (Madison: The State Historical Society of Wisconsin, 1948), p. 380. Interestingly, Dr. Hirshbuehl's cases were all in towns adjacent to Milwaukee. Though most of his patients lived in Bayview, Hirshbuehl did attend a few births in other suburban towns around Milwaukee. However, he never attended a woman living in the city.

10. Martin served as Commissioner of Health for Milwaukee from 1881 to 1890 (Still, *Milwaukee*, p. 385, n. 50). Judith Walzer Leavitt found that he was the only homeopathic physician ever to serve as health commissioner, and that neither the regular medical establishment nor the German members of the city council supported his appointment. See Leavitt, *The Healthiest City: Milwaukee and the Politics of Health Reform* (Princeton: Princeton University Press, 1982), p. 50.

11. As Figures 7.1 and 7.2 show, not every doctor in Milwaukee took on obstetrical cases, and many doctors who did took only a very few per year. For statistical reasons, "busy doctors" were defined as physicians who had attended at least ten births during some period in the thirty-six sampled months between 1870 and 1920. (The years sampled were 1873, 1877, 1880, 1885, 1890, 1895, 1900, 1905, 1910, 1915, and 1920.) No physician practiced during all of the sampled years, so the monthly average was higher than the simple division of ten births by thirty-six months.

12. The index for 1880 ranged from 0.000 to 0.714. The locality index, which was also used in Chapter 4 to assess the geographic limits of urban midwife practice, measured the number of wards a practitioner traveled from his or her own ward to attend a birth. The locality indices were constructed by weighting the number of deliveries by the distance from the attendant's home ward. Thus, a birth was weighted by zero if it occurred in the attendant's home ward, by one if it was in a contiguous ward, and so on. The sum of the weighted births was then divided by the total number of births to arrive at a weighted average. A mean locality index for the entire group practicing in a given year was determined for each of the three years. For "busy physicians," this figure translated into an average attendance at about 28 births per year, or about 2.3 deliveries per month. The mean for the 253 Milwaukee physicians identified as busy physicians was 27.81, with a standard deviation of 23.39. The minimum number was 6 births per year; the maximum was 175. To identify changes over time, I then chose three years (1880, 1900, and 1920) and computed locality indices for each busy physician practicing in that year. For 1880, the mean was based on indices calculated for six of the eleven busy doctors of 1880. For five physicians, indices could not be calculated because of the lack of patient address data in the birth records.

13. Five doctors (C. H. Lewis, E. W. Kellogg, H. S. Piggins, E. J. Purtell, and J. N. Rock) attended between 22 and 26 births in a three-month period. Most obstetricians consider a specialty practice to begin at the level of 10 births per month.

14. Polk's *Medical and Surgical Register of the U.S.* (1900), p. 1880, listed Fish as a Fellow of the American Association of Obstetrics and Gynecology.

15. The variance around the mean was very small; most doctors had an index greater than one, but less than two.

16. No correlation could be found between locality indices and the size of an obstetrical practice (the correlation coefficient between the locality index for each physician and the number of deliveries made by each doctor was 0.0577).

17. Dr. E. W. Kellogg, on the other hand, lived in the fifth ward on the south side, but six of his twenty-six births were across town in the northwest part of the city. However, Dr. James Williamson, who also lived in the fifth ward, oversaw only three births in this period, and he too traveled across town to his patients.

18. Paul Starr notes that the transportation revolution helped to expand the geographic limits of city practice. See Starr, *The Social Transformation of American Medicine: The Rise of a Sovereign Profession and the Making of a Vast Industry* (New York: Basic Books, 1982), p. 70. The rapid physical expansion of many American cities and the change from the "walking city" of the mid-nineteenth century to the "streetcar suburbs" of the late nineteenth and early twentieth centuries undoubtedly contributed to the expansion of physician practice. Sam Bass Warner's study of Boston was the first to examine the relationship between the growth of cities and the development of public transportation. See Warner's *Streetcar Suburbs: The Process of Growth in Boston, 1870–1900* (Cambridge: Harvard University Press, 1962). Roger D. Simon examined this process in Milwaukee in "The City-Building Process: Housing and Services in New Milwaukee Neighborhoods, 1880–1910," *Transactions of the American Philosophical Society* 68, pt. 5 (1978). In Milwaukee, electric trolley lines replaced horse-drawn trollies in 1890. The convenience of the new trollies was lauded in an 1891 *Milwaukee Journal* article, which noted that a person could now go across the city and back again within one hour (*Milwaukee Journal,* September 12, 1891, cited by Still, *Milwaukee,* p. 370). Roger Simon's study of Milwaukee's public transit system shows, however, that as late as 1910, though there were extensive streetcar routes all over the city, none crossed the Menomenee River Valley, which separated the north and south wards of Milwaukee (Roger David Simon, "The Expansion of an Industrial City: Milwaukee, 1880–1910," Ph.D. diss., University of Wisconsin, Madison, 1971, p. 162).

19. Guenter B. Risse points out that automobiles helped some physicians in the early twentieth century to triple the number of house calls they made in a day. See Risse, "From Horse and Buggy to Automobile and Telephone: Medical Practice in Wisconsin, 1848–1930," in Ronald L. Numbers and Judith Walzer Leavitt, eds., *Wisconsin Medicine: Historical Perspectives* (Madison: University of Wisconsin Press, 1981), p. 38.

20. By 1920, the average size of a physician's obstetrical practice had increased substantially to an average of between 4.5 and 5.0 births per month. A one-way ANOVA showed significant differences among the means of 1900–1905 versus 1920 (f-ratio = 5.825, f-probability = 0.00001). A Scheffe multiple range test showed significant differences between the means for 1920 and 1900 and 1920 and 1905. The increase in the mean number of deliveries per month was related more to the historical period than to the specific time the physician began to practice. Thus, the size of the obstetrical practice for each cohort increased after 1900, from about 2.5 to 5.0. For each cohort, the 95 percent confidence levels were as follows:

Cohort	Mean no. of babies per month	95% confidence for mean
1873	1.951	1.2254–2.6765
1877	1.2745	0.8628–1.6862
1880	1.4771	1.1434–1.8107
1885	2.3395	1.5634–3.1157
1890	1.7190	1.3037–2.1342
1895	3.0973	2.3593–3.8354
1900	2.4211	2.0806–2.7615
1905	2.9396	2.3996–3.4796
1910	3.1184	2.5888–3.6479
1915	4.1333	3.1538–5.1129
1920	4.8958	3.9022–5.8895

A one-way analysis of variance showed significant differences among the means for each cohort. However, due to the problem of heterogenous variances, a nonparametric Kruskal-Wallis test was used to determine significant differences among the average number of babies delivered per cohort. It showed a chi-square of 70.44, with a significance of 0.00001. Rather than being related to a specific cohort, the increase in the size of a practice was part of a general historical trend for all physicians. With the exception of 1873, for each of the years I sampled, there was an increase in the mean number of deliveries for every physician in practice that year, regardless of cohort. Thus, all doctors in 1920, regardless of the year that they began practice, were attending an average of about 4.5 to 5.0 births per month.

21. As noted later in the chapter, by 1920, some births in Milwaukee were taking place in hospitals. For this analysis of the geographic extent of physicians' obstetrical practice, the parents' residence is the primary concern, not where the birth actually took place. Locality indices were calculated based on the distance from the physician's home or office to the patient's home, regardless of where the woman delivered. As I wished to analyze the effect of neighborhood, and thus the possible social relationship between physician and patient, the site of the actual birth was not crucial for this analysis. The birth certificates for 1920 noted if the birth took place in a hospital as well as the parents' residence.

22. Sydney Halpern, in her analysis of the growth of pediatrics as a medical specialty, argues that the rise of medical specialties in America is a variant on the social science definition of professionalism. She then characterizes professionalization in terms of medical institutions, arguing that freestanding professions and medical specialties established occupational institutions to control recruitment and practice, structured markets for the delivery of services, competed among themselves for status and resources, and served as a means for collective upward mobility. Sydney A. Halpern, *American Pediatrics: The Social Dynamics of Professionalism, 1880–1980* (Berkeley: University of California Press, 1988), pp. 4–9. See also Rosemary Stevens, "The Changing Idea of a Medical Specialty," *Transactions and Studies of the College of Physicians of Philadelphia* 5 (1980): 159–177.

23. See John Harley Warner, *The Therapeutic Perspective: Medical Practice, Knowledge, and Identity in America, 1820–1885* (Cambridge: Harvard University Press, 1986), esp. Chapter 9, "Cui Bono?", pp. 258–284. Regina Markell Morantz-Sanchez

notes that women physicians had consciously adopted this more holistic idea of medical practice in the nineteenth century, and that by the early twentieth century, many decried the rise of specialism as leaving out the humane qualities they expected of physicians. See Morantz-Sanchez, *Sympathy and Science: Women Physicians in American Medicine* (New York: Oxford University Press, 1985), esp. Chapter 9, "Hopes Unfulfilled: Women Physicians and the Social Transformation of American Medicine," pp. 232–265.

24. Both the data from my study as well as current research show that most physicians consider ten deliveries or more per month to constitute an obstetrical specialty practice. Within the four counties, 1,067 physicians averaged 1.330 deliveries per month (1.00 standard deviation, 0.055 standard error). Only 1 percent of the physicians delivered about 10 births per month (value = 9.333). These numbers correspond to current findings on the average number of deliveries per month by family practitioners and obstetricians. At one busy, but representative, private hospital in Alabama, for example, obstetricians delivered an average of 10.83 babies per month (telephone conversation with Barbara Traylor, Director of Public Affairs, St. Vincent's Hospital, Birmingham, Alabama, August 1993). A survey of physicians published in 1992 showed that general and family practitioners attended an average of 0.9 vaginal deliveries per month (standard error of 0.1). Physicians who identified themselves as specializing in obstetrics and gynecology reported that they attended an average of 11.0 vaginal deliveries per month, with the median at 10 (standard error for mean 0.7). Fewer ob-gyn specialists reported doing cesarean sections, with an average of 3.7 per month (standard error of 0.6). See Martin L. Gonzalez, ed. *Physician Marketplace Statistics, 1992* (Chicago: Center for Health Policy Research, American Medical Association, 1992), table 24, p. 36.

25. Arthur Tenney Holbrook, "The First Twenty-five Years of the Milwaukee Surgical Society," manuscript read before the Society, November 5, 1951, unnumbered p. 2. Arthur Tenney Holbrook papers, Archives Division, State Historical Society of Wisconsin, Madison, Wisconsin.

26. L. H. Pelton, "Too Early Specialization?" *Wisconsin Medical Journal* 22 (1923–24): 446. Dr. Pelton was from Waupaca, Wisconsin.

27. Rosemary Stevens has argued that surgery, the earliest modern medical specialty, was the first place where the "delineation between a general practitioner and a specialist became a matter of acute concern." With the growth of hospitals, more general practitioners began doing surgery. Better trained surgeons deplored the lack of skill shown by these general practitioners, and they sought to establish their right to determine who should practice surgery (Stevens, *American Medicine,* 50.

28. Charles E. Rosenberg, *The Care of Strangers: The Rise of America's Hospital System* (New York: Basic Books, 1987), p. 169–173. Paul Starr argues that by the second and third decades of the twentieth century, if a physician wished to practice surgery, he or she would achieve the most success first by meeting the academic credentials imposed by the American College of Surgeons, and then joining with the College in promoting its goals (Starr, *Social Transformation of American Medicine,* pp. 177, 222).

29. Information on specialty interest was obtained from the American Medical Association, *American Medical Directory* (1921), pp. 1597–1603. A number of physicians not listed in Table 7.1 indicated in these directories that they were either interested or actually specializing in obstetrics, yet their actual practice, as measured

through the birth certificates, was far smaller than many of the physicians noted in Table 7.1. In the 1916 AMA *Directory,* for example, eighteen Milwaukee physicians indicated that they were full- or part-time obstetrical specialists, and Walter Darling indicated that he had limited his practice to this specialty. Walter Darling's maternity practice, however, was not large. I did not pick him up in this study until 1920, when he oversaw thirteen births in a three-month period.

30. For membership in specialty societies, see the listing "Members of Special Societies: Surgery, Gynecology, Obstetrics, and Anesthesia (Wisconsin)," *American Medical Directory* (1921), p. 93. Care should be used in defining specialists in terms of their membership in specialty societies. Neither Joseph B. DeLee nor J. Whitridge Williams, both eminent figures in the development of obstetrics in the early twentieth century, belonged in 1921 to the American Association of Obstetricians and Gynecologists. Indeed, they showed more interest in gynecological surgery. Dr. DeLee belonged to two gynecological societies and the American College of Surgeons (ibid., p. 80), and Dr. Williams belonged to the American Gynecological Society and the American College of Surgeons (ibid., p. 82). R. W. Roethke began his practice in Milwaukee in 1912, and in 1914, he joined the Marquette Medical College as their chief of gynecology and obstetrics. See W. G. Bruce, *History of Milwaukee, City and County,* 3 vols. (Chicago: S. J. Clarke, 1922), vol. 2, p. 228. G. W. Hipke was Professor of Obstetrics at the Wisconsin College of Physicians and Surgeons and one of the founders of the Milwaukee Maternity Hospital in 1906. By 1914 he was serving as the hospital's obstetrician-in-chief, with four associate and six assistant obstetricians. The hospital was established along the lines of Joseph B. DeLee's clinic in Chicago, primarily to train physicians to do outpatient deliveries. The hospital operated a dispensary to attract prenatal patients, most of whom would be delivered at home. Even in 1914, the hospital had only thirteen beds, and the organization attended to 268 obstetrical cases. See Louis Frederick Frank, *The Medical History of Milwaukee, 1834–1914* (Milwaukee: Germania Publishing Co., 1915), pp. 167–168; also Editor, "The Wisconsin Maternity Hospital," *Wisconsin Medical Journal* 4 (1905–6): 481–482 (this hospital was actually the Milwaukee Maternity Hospital). Neither Dr. Roethke nor Dr. Hipke showed up in the sample as delivering ten or more cases per month until 1920.

31. Only two of twenty-nine physicians listed in Milwaukee as obstetric specialists in the 1921 *American Medical Directory* limited their practice solely to obstetrics. The two were Dr. Cecil Lawhorn and Dr. James S. Thomas. The data on practice did not show high numbers of deliveries for either of these physicians, but an analysis of their training showed that both had spent a considerable amount of time in hospital training. (Lawhorn had 36 months, Thomas had 18; the mean for the group of 164 physicians in my sample trained between 1910 and 1919 was 6.88 months.)

32. Starr argues that in the period between 1870 and 1910, "hospital appointments became more valuable as hospitals became indispensable for surgical practice and specialization advanced" (*Social Transformation of American Medicine,* p. 163). Hospitals, he argues, also encouraged the development of specialties by helping specialists to lower their indirect costs and to concentrate on providing services that offered the highest return (ibid., p. 77). Charles E. Rosenberg argues that the medical specialties of the twentieth century grew out of the more informal relationships in nineteenth-century hospitals. Indeed, he states, many of the specialty boards "mandated and formalized already well-established patterns of training, staffing, and practice" that

had existed in the nineteenth century. (Rosenberg, *The Care of Strangers,* p. 175). While this is undoubtedly true in the more elite academic centers of the East, access to hospital practice in Milwaukee seemed much more democratic.

33. The licenses for 18 of the 21 physicians in this sample were used for *t*-tests for significant differences between them and the other physicians in the sample. All tests for significant differences in the mean years of education and the number of months in the hospital were negative (for the mean number of years of medical lectures: mean for obstetricians = 3.67, for all other doctors = 3.69, $t = -0.15$, 19.08 *df,* 2-tail probability = 0.883; for months of hospital training: mean for obstetricians = 5.61, mean for all other doctors = 7.22, $t = -0.55$, 774 *df,* 2-tail probability = 0.609). When the group of other doctors was narrowed to include just Milwaukee physicians, the results were the same (mean number of years of medical lectures: obstetricians = 3.67, Milwaukee doctors = 3.71, $t = -0.27$, 20.05 *df,* 2-tail probability = 0.788; for months of hospital training: obstetricians = 5.61, Milwaukee doctors = 7.1, $t = -0.45$, 540 *df,* 2-tail probability = 0.653). The only significant difference for this group was their date of graduation (mean for obstetricians = 1902, for all other doctors in sample = 1897, $t = 2.64$, 20.11 *df,* 2-tail probability = 0.015). However, when these practitioners were compared with others who registered after 1900, there were no significant differences in the mean years of education or months of hospital training.

34. Frank's *Medical History of Milwaukee* notes at least five hospitals in 1913–14 that accepted maternity patients. Thirty-four physicians were named as being on the obstetrical staff of these hospitals, but only four of these doctors turned up in my 1915 birth sample as having attended ten cases or more per month (Frank, *The Medical History of Milwaukee,* pp. 149, 152, 154, 167, 173).

35. Polk's *Medical and Surgical Register of the U.S.* (1900) lists seven Milwaukee physicians, including Dr. Edmund Fish, who listed himself as a "Fellow of the American Association of Obstetrics and Gynecology" (p. 1830). In the 1921 AMA *Directory,* twenty-nine Milwaukee doctors listed themselves as full- or part-time obstetrical specialists; seven of these doctors appeared in my data for 1920 as having delivered ten or more babies per month.

36. John Warner argues that epistemological changes were at the heart of the most important shifts in nineteenth century medical practice. See Warner, *Therapeutic Perspective.*

37. Judith Waltzer Leavitt, *Brought to Bed: Childbearing in America, 1750–1950* (New York: Oxford University Press, 1986), esp. Chapter 4 "Only a Woman Can Know: The Role of Gender in the Birthing Room," pp. 87–115.

38. While Sydney Halpern's study of pediatrics, like the previously cited studies of specialization, emphasizes the role of institutions, she goes beyond the others to stress the need to look at changing patterns of labor that impel professionalization. "Collectivities," or groups of practitioners, she argues, came together as the result of changes in the patterns of work. Professionalization, she insists, was, "at least in part, a codification of emerging patterns of labor" (Halpern, *American Pediatrics,* pp. 19, 23).

39. At least two Polish-surnamed midwives claimed that Dr. Wasielewski had provided some of their training. See license applications of Jadwiga Kuzminska and Frances Jahnz, Board of Medical Examiners, Midwife File, Series 1611, Archives Division, Wisconsin State Historical Society, Madison, Wisconsin (hereafter Midwife

File, WSHS). Wasielewski also signed nine midwife licenses as either the first or second physician.

40. Information on Dr. Wasielewski's patients comes from Birth Records, Milwaukee County, May–July 1910, 1915, and 1920. Filed with State of Wisconsin Department of Health and Human Services Vital Records Office, Madison, Wisconsin.

41. Starr, *Social Transformation of American Medicine,* p. 167.

42. Wasielewski, Wagner, and five other physicians began this work in 1911. For a good description of the politics of this commission, see Leavitt, *The Healthiest City,* pp. 216–228.

43. Frank, *Medical History of Milwaukee,* pp. 158–159; 173.

44. The Polish Physicians and Dentists Association was still active in 1946. The sources differ slightly on its founding members. John J. Kazmierowski, credits Dr. Karol (Karl) Wagner, together with Dr. J. Rozmarynowski, a dentist, with forming the organization in 1913. See Kazmierowski's "Our Medical Profession," in Thaddeus Borun, comp., *We, the Milwaukee Poles: The History of Milwaukeans of Polish Descent and a Record of Their Contributions to the Greatness of Milwaukee* (Milwaukee: Nowiny Publishing Co., 1946), p. 85. However, Wasielewski's biographer in *Wisconsin: Stability, Progress, Beauty* (5 vols., Chicago: Lewis Publishing Co., 1946), credits him with founding this society (vol. 5, pp. 17–18). It is likely, given Wagner's senior position in the community, that he was the guiding force behind setting up the society. (Wagner was described as one of the most influential Polish men in Milwaukee, meriting a separate biography in the Milwaukee Polish community's history in 1946. See Miecislaus Haiman, "Dr. Karol Wagner," in Boren, *We, the Milwaukee Poles,* p. 58.) However, Wasielewski was an active practitioner in the community by this time and probably was involved (Kazmierowski, "Our Medical Profession," in Boren, *We, the Milwaukee Poles,* p. 85). Whatever his role in founding the Polish Physicians' and Dentists' Association, Wasielewski was more active in the Polish community than he was in Milwaukee's institutional medical circles. During the First World War, he was involved in helping to recruit soldiers from Milwaukee's Polish-American community. He was also active in obtaining relief for Poland. Information on Dr. Wasielewski is taken from his obituary, "Arrange Rites for Physician," *Milwaukee Journal,* February 4, 1937, and Kazmierowski, "Our Medical Profession," in Boren, *We, the Milwaukee Poles,* pp. 83–84. Wasielewski's son Thaddeus became actively involved in political life in the city, and was elected to the U.S. House of Representatives in 1938 (Still, *Milwaukee,* p. 468).

45. Karl Wagner signed at least twenty different midwife licenses; Frank Wasielewski trained two midwives and signed at least nine midwife licenses. A. A. Krygier signed four licenses, and S. L. Krzysko signed one. Midwife File, WSHS.

46. Though Drs. Wasielewski and Wagner were listed on the obstetrical staff of Misericordia Hospital, not one of the births attributed to these doctors in this study took place in a hospital. In 1920, the three other doctors of Polish background in this group each delivered only one baby in a hospital.

47. These second-generation immigrant professionals who practiced in their own neighborhoods challenge some assumptions that historians and sociologists have made concerning professionals in the Progressive Era. A number of scholars have emphasized that the demographic composition of the professional middle class in the Progressive Era was native-born, white, and Protestant. Harold Wilensky's pioneering work on the problems of defining professionals asserted that one of their distin-

guishing characteristics was their upper-middle class and Protestant background. See Harold L. Wilensky, "The Professionalization of Everyone?" *American Journal of Sociology* 70 (1964): 151. Many historians have adopted this model, and indeed many studies of the Progressive Era have argued that it was this group's anxieties about status that led to the reforms and the excesses of Progressivism. Paul Boyer makes this argument explicitly in his discussion of the roots of Progressivism. See Paul S. Boyer, *Urban Masses and Moral Order in America, 1820–1920* (Cambridge: Harvard University Press, 1978). See also Robert H. Wiebe, *The Search for Order, 1877–1920* (New York: Hill and Wang, 1967).

48. Even Walter Channing, the first instructor in obstetrics at Harvard Medical School in Boston in the early nineteenth century, delivered very few babies per month. Though he had had extensive training in obstetrics at Edinburgh, founded the Boston Lying-In Hospital, and was one of the founders of the *New England Journal of Medicine and Surgery,* Channing attended only between ten and thirty deliveries per year. See Amalie M. Kass, "The Obstetrical Case Book of Walter Channing, 1811–1822," *Bulletin of the History of Medicine* 67 (1993): 494–523. Like other sociologists of the professions, Paul Starr has argued that medical institutions helped to promote a collegial relationship between physicians. This collegial relationship replaced the physician-patient relationship as a prime factor in determining a physician's success. See Starr, *Social Transformation of American Medicine,* pp. 168, 362. JoAnne Brown argues that it is not enough to know the material conditions under which an emerging profession labored. Instead, she maintains, the language professionals used to justify their special status explains how these conditions were translated into consciousness. See Brown, "Professional Language: Words that Succeed," *Radical History Review* 34 (1986): 33–51.

49. Dr. Graettinger, who had trained a number of German midwives in Milwaukee, served as chairman of the Committee in 1890. See State Medical Society of Wisconsin, "Officers and Members for 1890–91," *Transactions* 24 (1890–91): x. Dr. Noer became the chair of the Obstetrics Committee in 1900. See State Medical Society of Wisconsin, "Committees," *Transactions* 34 (1900–01): 13. In an 1898 paper, "The Midwifery Question," Noer discussed the adamant opposition by some obstetricians to midwives, but argued that the situation was different in Wisconsin, where families were large and immigrant women were "in the habit of employing midwives" and therefore "do not take kindly to the idea of being legally compelled to employ a physician." Indeed, he saw the "educated midwife" as an aid "not only to the people, but to the physician also." Noer, "The Midwifery Question," *Transactions of the State Medical Society of Wisconsin* 32 (1898): 389–391. Noer's comments on requiring hospitalization for all births were found in "Comments" to W. F. McCabe, "Obstetrical Responsibility during Gestation," *Wisconsin Medical Journal* 5 (1906–7): 601. Interestingly, even a Milwaukee physician thought that Noer's idea was "a condition of the future . . . far in the distance" (H. Sylvester, ibid., p. 601).

50. See Rosenberg, *The Care of Strangers,* esp. pp. 164–165 for a discussion of the role of the hospital at the turn of the twentieth century in promoting physician prestige. Rosenberg also provides an example of how this entire system worked for one ambitious turn-of-the century medical graduate in "Making it in Urban Medicine: A Career in the Age of Scientific Medicine," *Bulletin of the History of Medicine* 64 (1990): 163–186.

51. Information on Dr. Hipke was found in several obituaries for his wife, Clara

B. Hipke. See "$16,500 Given to Set Up M. U. Obstetrics Library," *Milwaukee Journal,* January 6, 1948; "Establish Library in Honor of Late Clara B. Hipke," unidentified Wisconsin newspaper clipping found in Dr. Alfred Belitz papers, Manuscript Collection 56 PB, Archives Division, Wisconsin State Historical Society, Madison. Hipke was listed in the 1904 edition of Polk's *Medical Register and Directory of North America* as a Professor of Obstetrics. See 8th ed. (1904), p. 2002.

52. Clara Hipke, it appears, was instrumental in founding this hospital, and she remained an active fund-raiser until her death in 1938. As president of the Maternity Hospital and Dispensary Association, she also led a fight for the passage in Wisconsin of the enabling legislation for Sheppard-Towner and the Wisconsin "silver nitrate" law ("$16,500 Given" and "Establish Library").

53. The average for all four academic doctors in 1905 was 2.42.

54. See Chapter 5 for a discussion of the turmoil in medical education in Milwaukee. See also Ronald L. Numbers, "A Note on Medical Education in Wisconsin," Numbers and Leavitt, *Wisconsin Medicine,* pp. 177–184.

55. Rosemary Stevens notes that surveys of practicing physicians in the first decades of the twentieth century found that as many as 35 percent of medical school graduates were full-time specialists within six years of graduating from medical school. Young physicians in these early decades especially eschewed general practice: a survey of 1920 medical school graduates of class A medical schools found that almost three-quarters of them (74 percent) intended to restrict their practice to some specialty. Stevens, *American Medicine,* p. 147, n. 41. Cautionary note about specialties is found in the AMA *American Medical Directory* (1921), p. 7.

56. Six physicians on the 1920 list of large practice obstetricians also claimed specialty interest in the 1921 *Directory,* but though three of the five Polish physicians had the most active practices in 1920, not one of the five made this claim.

57. By the early twentieth century, the German community in Milwaukee was in decline; in 1884, for example, German-language newspapers had nearly twice the circulation of their rival English-language ones, but by 1910, English-language newspapers outsold German ones by a three to one margin. See Robert C. Nesbit, *Wisconsin: A History* (Madison: University of Wisconsin Press, 1973), pp. 347–348. Despite the Americanization of the press, however, many Milwaukee residents still identified with a German background and, as noted in Chapter 5, many of the physicians in this sample had parents or grandparents from Germany.

58. I found 25 of the 29 physicians from this list among those in the sample of Milwaukee physician-assisted births. Of these physicians, 24 appeared in the 1920 sample; of these 24 doctors, 21 used the hospital at least once, and 10 of them used the hospital for at least half of their patients. Among the large practice physicians, however, only 2 primarily used the hospital.

59. See Dr. Noer's comments above. Judith Walzer Leavitt points out that popular women's magazines helped to convince middle-class women that hospitals could offer them science and safety. See Leavitt, *Brought to Bed,* Chapter 7, "Alone among Strangers: Birth Moves to the Hospital," pp. 171–195.

60. For information on Dr. Roethke's training, see his license, filed in 1912 (Board of Medical Examiners, Physician Licenses, Series 1606, Archives Division, Wisconsin State Historical Society, Madison, Wisconsin). His postgraduate training was noted in his biographical entry in Bruce, *History of Milwaukee,* vol. 2, p. 228. He was described in this biography as "one of the eminent specialists in this field [obstetrics]

in the state." Information on Roethke's professional affiliations can be found in the AMA, *American Medical Directory* (1921), p. 1602.

61. In the sampled months of 1920, Roethke delivered forty of his forty-nine patients in hospitals.

62. Information on patients is from Birth Records, Milwaukee County, May–July 1920.

63. For a laudatory biography, see W. G. Bruce, "Rudolph Walter Roethke, M.D.," in W. G. Bruce, *History of Milwaukee, City and County* 3 vols. (Chicago: S.J. Clarke, 1922), vol. 2, pp. 228–231. By 1931, he was listed in private practice, but he was noted as being the author of *Medical Student's Outline of Obstetrics* and *Nurse's Outlines of Obstetrics*. See biography in *A Biographical Directory of Practicing Members of the Medical Profession in the United States and Canada* (Minneapolis: The Midwest Co., 1931), p. 1408.

64. Roethke's article from this meeting was printed and reprinted in two consecutive volumes of the *Wisconsin Medical Journal*. The discussion was printed only in vol. 18. R. W. Roethke, "Indications for Davis Caesarian Section," *Wisconsin Medical Journal* 17 (1918–19): 359–361; 18 (1919–20): 212–215. Quote is from vol. 18, p. 215.

65. Leavitt argues that urban, middle-class women began to call in physicians for their confinements by the end of the eighteenth and into the nineteenth centuries because they believed that physician obstetrics offered increased safety (Leavitt, *Brought to Bed*, pp. 79–80). See also Sylvia D. Hoffert, *Private Matters: American Attitudes toward Childbearing and Infant Nurture in the Urban North, 1800–1860* (Urbana: University of Illinois Press, 1989).

66. Walter T. Dannreuther, "The American Board of Obstetrics and Gynecology: Its Organization, Function, and Objectives," *Journal of the American Medical Association* 96 (1931): 797–798; quoted by Stevens, *American Medicine and the Public Interest*, p. 202.

67. Stevens, *American Medicine and the Public Interest*, p. 203.

68. J. P. Greenhill, ed., *Yearbook of Obstetrics and Gynecology*, (Chicago: Year Book Medical Publishers) 1936; quoted by Stevens, *American Medicine and the Public Interest*, p. 203. Under rules in place until 1942, a doctor who limited his or her practice solely to obstetrics and then took either an examination or had postgraduate training in obstetrics could qualify for Board membership. Dr. Roethke could have qualified under these criteria, but for some reason he chose not to. He was listed in the AMA *Directory* through at least 1950 as limiting his practice to obstetrics and gynecology.

69. The Verein Deutscher Aerzte was founded in Milwaukee in 1883 and was limited to those possessing a German medical degree. The purpose of the organization was to promote scientific discourse and "professional interests" which, given the ethnic restrictions on membership, were defined in cultural terms. Indeed, the "professional interests" included the promotion of a German identity. A picture in Frank's *Medical History of Milwaukee* showed members of the organization standing with a member of the German royal family on an American visit. The organization was disbanded in 1907, when the society realized that it could not add more members. Though Alois Graettinger, who trained midwives in the late nineteenth century, was a member, none of the active obstetricians found in my study was listed as a member (Frank, *Medical History of Milwaukee*, p. 128). Though the Polish Physicians' and Dentists' Association was cited in Borun as being active as late as 1946, by this date

it was undoubtedly a purely social organization (Kazmierowski, "Our Medical Profession," in Borun, *We, the Milwaukee Poles,* p. 85). Though the criteria for Board membership was established so as to include physicians who had been in practice prior to the establishment of the Board, most of the Milwaukee doctors in this study did not take on Board membership. A check in the 1939 *Directory of Medical Specialists* revealed that of the eight Milwaukee Board-certified obstetricians, only one, Julius Sure, had received his medical degree in the early twentieth century (1903). The other seven specialists were younger men. However, four of the thirteen 1920 large practice obstetricians continued to list their specialty interest in the AMA *Directory* as late as 1940. See Paul Titus, ed., *Directory of Medical Specialists,* (New York: Columbia University Press, 1940), pp. 335–336; American Medical Association, *Directory, 1940* (Chicago, 1940), pp. 1857–1866.

70. A number of displaced persons with foreign medical degrees applied for Wisconsin licenses in the 1940s, and the Board turned them all down. Defining an acceptable medical degree as one only from an American or Canadian school, the Board refused to license one physician who had an M.D. and a Ph.D. from the Kaiser Wilhelm Institute in Berlin, and had done research at the Rockefeller Institute in New York. See Board of Medical Examiners, "Newspaper Clippings about a D. P. Doctor, 1948," Series 70/0/15, Box No. 1, Archives Division, Wisconsin State Historical Society, Madison, Wisconsin. There were stories about three different doctors in this file. My thanks to Joanne Hohler for bringing these to my attention.

71. National studies show that about 30 percent of all American maternity cases in 1930 took place in hospitals, but studies of individual urban areas showed that hospital births ranged from 50 to more than 80 percent. See Rosemary Stevens, *In Sickness and in Wealth: American Hospitals in the Twentieth Century* (New York: Basic Books, 1989), p. 382, n. 1; also Joyce Antler and Daniel M. Fox, "The Movement towards a Safe Maternity: Physician Accountability in New York City, 1915–1940" in Judith Walzer Leavitt and Ronald L. Numbers, eds., *Sickness and Health in America: Readings in the History of Medicine and Public Health,* 2nd ed., rev. (Madison: University of Wisconsin Press, 1985), p. 493.

72. Stevens, *In Sickness and in Wealth,* pp. 113–114.

73. Myron Wegman, "Annual Survey of Vital Statistics, 1974," *Pediatrics* 56 (1975): 960–966, quoted by Doris Haire, *The Cultural Warping of Childbirth: A Special Report* (Hillside, N.J.: International Childbirth Education Association, 1976), p. 5.

74. Haire, *Cultural Warping of Childbirth,* postscript, p. 36.

Conclusion

1. When she was thirty-five years old and a new graduate of the Wisconsin College of Midwifery, Zoladkiewicz registered with the State Board of Medical Examiners in 1912. Board of Medical Examiners, Midwife File, Series 1611, Archives Division, Wisconsin State Historical Society, Madison, Wisconsin; hereafter referred to as Midwife File, WSHS. Zoladkiewicz was listed in the Midwives section of Wright's *Milwaukee City Directory* (Milwaukee: Alfred G. Wright) from 1920 through 1945.

2. In 1950, two women were listed in the AMA *Directory* in Milwaukee as being obstetrical specialists. While there had been a female Board-certified specialist in Madison as early as 1939, there was not one listed in Milwaukee until 1951, when

one woman was listed. She was one of only three Board-certified women in the state in that year. American Board for Medical Specialties, *Directory of Medical Specialists* (Chicago: A. N. Marquis Co., 1951), pp. 484–485.

3. See Chapter 7 for a discussion of Dr. Wasielewski's training and practice. In the sampled years of Wasielewski's practice, the overwhelming majority of his maternity patients were Polish immigrant women from blue-collar families. Wasielewski was also active in the child welfare movement in Milwaukee's South Side. See Judith Walzer Leavitt, *The Healthiest City: Milwaukee and the Politics of Health Reform* (Princeton: Princeton University Press, 1982), n. 24, p. 225 (note that his name is spelled "Wasiolewski").

4. Birth Records, Price and Trempealeau County, 1920, 1930. Filed at the State of Wisconsin Department of Health and Human Services Vital Records Office, Madison, Wisconsin.

5. The listings in the Madison city directories had been declining throughout the second decade of the twentieth century; only three midwives were listed in 1914. See "Midwives," classified listings, Angell's *Madison, Wisconsin City Directory, 1916* (G.R. Angell Co., 1916). Mrs. Mary Alsheimer was the only person to advertise as a midwife in Madison in 1919, the last year any Madison midwife did so. (She birthed five babies in 1920.) See "Midwives," classified listings, Wright's *Madison City Directory, 1919* (Milwaukee, Wisconsin: Wright Directory Co., 1919; also Birth Records, Dane County, 1920. Filed with Dane County Vital Records Office, City-County Building, Madison, Wisconsin.

6. See records for State Board of Medical Examiners, "Minutes," 1915–1935 (Microfilm), Series 1603, Archives Division, State Historical Society of Wisconsin, Madison, Wisconsin. At the January 8, 1924, meeting, three midwives appeared before the board to be allowed to take the examination in their native languages. It is unclear from the minutes if the tests were given in Polish, German, and Italian, but the women did receive their licenses. In 1928, a Racine midwife was tested by Dr. Brewer of the Board in a language other than English.

7. Though Cesario had petitioned the Board to give the examination in her native language, the Board agreed to give her a license if she would take the test in English. It is unclear how the examination was administered, but Cesario was licensed that afternoon (Board of Medical Examiners, "Minutes," June 26, 1922).

8. Board of Medical Examiners, "Minutes." Mary Mazurek's application was denied at the January 10, 1933, meeting, and Minnie P. Potter was turned down at the meeting on June 26, 1933. Cardinal was the last midwife in the state to receive a midwife license.

9. Many physician critics of midwives leveled this criticism in the early twentieth century. Two studies of midwife practice, one in Chicago and one in Massachusetts, showed widely varying numbers of midwives performing abortions. James Lincoln Huntington's survey of Massachusetts midwives estimated that only 5 percent of the midwives he investigated were suspected of performing abortions; see Huntington, "Midwives in Massachusetts," *Boston Medical and Surgical Journal* 167 (1912), p. 547. The Committee on Midwives' study of Chicago midwives, however, estimated that one-third of Chicago midwives had "criminal" practices; see "The Midwives of Chicago," *Journal of the American Medical Association* 50 (1908): 1348–1349.

10. Maria Polacek, a Milwaukee midwife, had her certificate of registration revoked in April 1932 when she was convicted of "producing a miscarriage." Minnie Went-

land's registration was revoked in 1933 when she was convicted of "performing an illegal operation" (Board of Medical Examiners, "Minutes"). Orsola Casoria's registration was revoked in 1937 when the Board learned she was charged with manslaughter; see State Board of Medical Examiners, Complaint and Revocation File— Midwives, Series 1873, Box 1, Archives Division, Wisconsin State Historical Society, Madison, Wisconsin. The subject of the relationship between midwives and abortion is a fascinating one. Though I did not find much evidence linking the midwives in my sample with abortions, Leslie Reagan has found that some Chicago midwives were performing abortions in addition to their regular birthing duties. See Leslie J. Reagan, "Midwives at Work: Providing Abortions," paper given at the 66th Annual Meeting of the American Association for the History of Medicine, May 14, 1993, Louisville, Kentucky.

11. Dr. George L. Gibbs, who was also convicted of practicing abortion in 1924, had been president of the village of Marshall, Wisconsin. His license was restored in 1924. Denying the charges or showing remorse and having many supporting letters seemed to sway the Board in favor of reinstatement. Those who dared to defend the practice did not have their licenses reinstated. For example, I. M. Brown, a New London physician, was convicted of providing abortions in 1935. Pleading guilty, he argued that someone should be doing it. His license was not reinstated. Information on the eleven doctors was taken from their medical licenses. Though the Board of Medical Examiners had a Complaint and Revocation file, it was not complete. But such information was recorded on the physician's license if he or she was accused or convicted of a crime, a fact that I noted as I went through the boxes of license files for the physicians in this study. As I examined every Wisconsin doctor's license filed between 1898 and 1930, I noted when a doctor was accused or convicted of providing an abortion. Among the eleven physicians I found was Fred Liefert. Liefert was one of the physicians in my Milwaukee sample of physicians and one of the ten busiest obstetricians in Milwaukee in 1920. In 1931, he was convicted of second degree manslaughter. He spent five years in jail in Milwaukee, yet his license was reinstated in 1936. See Board of Medical Examiners, Physician Licenses, Boxes 1898–1930, Series 1606, Archives Division, Wisconsin State Historical Society, Madison, Wisconsin.

12. Many midwives in traditional agricultural societies practiced this kind of folk medicine; indeed, they were the first practitioners outside of the family that a sick person might consult. For a good example in early nineteenth century America, see the description of Martha Ballard's medical work in Laurel Thatcher Ulrich, *A Midwife's Tale: The Life of Martha Ballard, Based on Her Diary, 1785–1812* (New York: Knopf, 1990), Chapter 1, "August 1787, 'Exceeding Dangerously Ill,' " pp. 36–71. Information on Josephine Krzyzanowska can be found in the Midwife File, WSHS; 1910 federal census; and Birth Records, Milwaukee County, 1900–1920, WSHS. Information on her prosecution for "Polish medicine" can be found in Board of Medical Examiners, Complaint and Revocation File—M.D.s, Series 1616, Archives Division, Wisconsin State Historical Society, Madison, Wisconsin.

13. In 1915, only 26 percent of babies in Milwaukee and 12.9 percent in the entire state were born with the aid of a midwife. Dorothy Reed Mendenhall, "Prenatal and Natal Conditions in Wisconsin," *Wisconsin Medical Journal* 15 (1917): 357.

14. The American Medical Association *AMA Directory* (Chicago: American Medical Association) for 1940 listed forty-two physicians in Milwaukee, one in Trempe-

aleau County, none in Price County, and twelve in Dane County. Only two of the doctors in Dane County were outside of Madison; and of the ten in Madison, four were professors of obstetrics and gynecology at the medical school (pp. 1857–1866). Drs. Roethke and Krygier, mentioned in the Chapter 7, were listed in the *Directory* of 1950. Lists of physicians who met Board certification requirements are found in *Directory of Medical Specialists, 1939* (New York: Columbia University Press, 1940), pp. 335–336; and *Directory of Medical Specialists, 1951* (Chicago: A.N. Marquis Co., 1951), pp. 484–485. Though Dr. Roethke remained listed as limiting his practice to obstetrics and gynecology, he never was Board certified.

15. Board of Health, Madison, Wisconsin, *Reports* (1924). The statewide figure was for cities with a population of over 10,000 U.S. Department of Commerce, Bureau of the Census, "Percent Resident Births . . . Hospitals . . . ," *Vital Statistics of the United States* (Washington, D.C., 1938), Part 2, Table Z, p. 15. By 1940, 55.8 percent of births nationally were in hospitals, and 90.8 percent of all births were physician-attended. However, like Wisconsin, the national figures for urban births were much different than those for rural ones: 76.0 percent of all urban women gave birth in hospitals in 1940, while 32.3 percent of rural women did. U.S. Department of Health, Education, and Welfare, Public Health Service, *Vital Statistics of the United States, 1950*, 3 vols. (Washington, D.C.: National Office of Vital Statistics, 1950), vol. 1, table 6.31, p. 95; table 6.32, p. 96.

16. For a good discussion of the interaction of the medical and the social concerns underlying the building of rural hospitals after 1920, see Rosemary Stevens, *In Sickness and in Wealth: American Hospitals in the Twentieth Century* (New York: Basic Books, 1989), pp. 119–125. Stevens finds that the proportion of counties in the United States that lacked hospitals had dropped from over 50 percent in 1920 to 40 percent in 1930 (p. 125).

17. Numbers of hospital births are taken from: U.S. Bureau of Commerce, Bureau of the Census, "Percent Resident Births and Recorded Births, Occurring in Hospitals, 1940," *Vital Statistics of the United States, 1940* (Washington, D.C., 1943), part II, table T, pp. 14–15. The number of hospitals was found in American Medical Association, *AMA Directory, 1940*, p. 1844–1847. There were at least six hospitals in Dane County, two in Trempealeau County, three in Price County, and ten in Milwaukee County. Note that these were general hospitals; the hospital in Phillips, for example, was a maternity home opened by a local physician in 1940 and run by a registered nurse until 1963. Centennial Committee, "Maternity Homes," *Centennial Phillips, Wisconsin* (Phillips, Wisconsin, 1976), pp. 170–171.

18. DeLee, "Progress towards Ideal Obstetrics," *American Journal of Obstetrics and Diseases of Women and Children* 73 (1916): 407–415.

19. DeLee, "The Prophylactic Forceps Operation," *American Journal of Obstetrics and Gynecology* 1 (1920–21): 34–44. A number of scholars have cited this article as one of the most influential statements on obstetrical technique in the first half of the twentieth century. Both Barbara Katz Rothman and Judith Walzer Leavitt argue that DeLee's article was extremely important in moving birth to the hospital. See Rothman, "Awake and Aware, or False Consciousness: The Cooption of Shelly Romalis, Childbirth Reform in America," in Shelly Romalis, ed., *Childbirth: Alternatives to Medical Control* (Austin: University of Texas Press, 1981), p. 150–151; Leavitt, *Brought to Bed: Childbearing in America, 1750–1950* (New York: Oxford University Press, 1986), pp. 179–180.

20. The figures are found in *Vital Statistics of the United States, 1950,* vol. 1, table 6.32, p. 96; and *Vital Statistics of the United States, 1960,* vol. 1, p. 11.

21. Many southern states did not begin to regulate midwifery until the years after World War I. South Carolina's law was typical. Passed in 1920, it required midwives to register with their local community. While nurses in South Carolina offered classes in hygiene to the mostly black midwives, states like Alabama merely kept lists of midwives. See Ruth A. Dodd, "Midwife Supervision in South Carolina," *Public Health Nurse* 12 (1920): 863–867. By the 1920s, with the aid of Sheppard-Towner funds, many southern states set up programs to help teach black midwives the rudiments of asepsis. In many cases, black nurses were recruited for this purpose. Eunice Rivers, for example, who later became famous for her participation in the Tuskegee syphilis experiment, began her nursing career in Macon County, Georgia, teaching maternity care to new mothers and educating the local midwives. In Mississippi, public health nurses supervised midwifery practice and were in charge of granting permits to practice. Throughout the 1930s and 1940s, administrative changes were made in how black midwives were supervised, but even in the 1950s, many southern states continued to work with black midwives even as they blamed them for the south's very high infant mortality rate. See Darlene Clark Hine, *Black Women in White: Racial Conflict and Cooperation in the Nursing Profession, 1890–1950* (Bloomington: Indiana University Press, 1989), pp. 154–155; Onnie Lee Logan as told to Katherine Clark, *Motherwit: An Alabama Midwife's Story* (New York: E. P. Dutton, 1989), pp. x–xi; and Rene M. Reeb, "Granny Midwives in Mississippi: Career and Birthing Practices," *Journal of Transcultural Nursing* 4 (1992): 18–27.

22. *Vital Statistics of the United States, 1950,* 3 vols. (Washington, D.C.: United States Department of Health, Education, and Welfare, Public Health Service, National Office of Vital Statistics), vol. 1, table 6.32, p. 96. I used the figures in this table labeled "non-white," as 90 percent of the births in this category were attributed to the category "Negro" (see description, p. 118).

23. *Vital Statistics of the United States,* 1960, vol. 1, p. 12; 1970, vol. 1, p. 33.

24. Logan, *Motherwit,* p. xiv.

25. More than one-fifth of all general hospitals in the United States in 1940 formally excluded black patients, and even the passage of the Hill-Burton legislation in the late 1940s did not force hospitals to accept black patients. In many areas of the southern United States, only the double impact of the Civil Rights Act of 1964 and the Medicare Legislation of 1965 forced hospitals to accept black patients (Stevens, *In Sickness and in Wealth,* pp. 175, 254).

26. *Childbirth without Fear* was published in the United States in 1944, and *Painless Childbirth* was published in 1956. The Lamaze method was introduced into the United States in 1959 by Marjorie Karmel, a woman who had gone to Paris to have her baby with Dr. Lamaze. See Karmel, *Thank You, Dr. Lamaze: A Mother's Experience in Painless Childbirth* (Philadelphia: Lippincott, 1959). Both Judith Walzer Leavitt (*Brought to Bed,* pp. 214–215) and Barbara Katz Rothman ("Awake and Aware," in Romalis, *Childbirth,* pp. 150–180) have argued that Dick-Read and Lamaze-type preparation were developed in the American context as efforts to reform hospital birthing practices.

27. Suzanne Arms and Adrienne Rich are among the many writers of the 1970s who noted the influence of the gender of the birth practitioner and advocated a more egalitarian, same-gender birth attendant. See Arms, *Immaculate Deception: A New*

Look at Women and Childbirth in America (Boston: Houghton Mifflin, 1975); and Rich, *Of Woman Born: Motherhood as Experience and Institution* (New York: Bantam Books, 1976), esp. Chapter 7, "Alienated Labor" pp. 149–182. Ina May Gaskin was one of the most influential of the counterculture authors of the 1970s. Her book, *Spiritual Midwifery,* became a best-seller and has sold well over 500,000 copies around the world. Ina May and the Farm Midwives, *Spiritual Midwifery* (Summertown, Tenn.: The Book Publishing Co., 1975). For a recent analysis, see Jessica Mitford, *The American Way of Birth* (New York: Dutton, 1992), pp. 197–207. Interestingly, Gaskin's description of the qualities needed by a midwife sounds very much like those required by early twentieth-century midwives: "a real midwife," says Gaskin, should be spiritual, compassionate, able to consider someone else's viewpoint, and "in her daily life take care of those around her." Gaskin's "spiritual midwife" was to "be married and have a solid, loving, honest relationship with her husband." She was to "have had a child naturally, and have a solid, loving relationship with her children." She was also to be "an avid student of physiology and medicine" (pp. 338–339).

28. The number of female Fellows of the American College of Obstetricians and Gynecologists has grown in recent years. In 1993, there were 8,115 women out of a total of 41,432 (19.6 percent); the number in Wisconsin was slightly higher, 59 out of 268 total members (22 percent). The number will rise as more junior physicians finish their residency training. In 1990–91, almost 49 percent of ob-gyn residents were women (Resource Center, American College of Obstetricians and Gynecologists, Washington, D.C.; Mitford, *American Way of Birth,* p. 102). Interestingly, neither the American College of Nurse-Midwives nor the American College of Obstetricians and Gynecologists could give me current numbers or percentages on the number of minority practitioners in their fields.

29. See Augusto Sarmiento, "Editorial: Orthopaedics at a Crossroads," *The Journal of Bone and Joint Surgery* 75-A (1993): 159–161. Sarmiento points out that many of the surgical specialties have become so fragmented into subspecialties that the group as a whole has lost political power. He notes that many policy experts have advocated limiting the number of residencies for specialist training and even that those who wish surgical specialist training pay for it themselves, much as they did with medical school. Orthopedists now face cost competition from podiatrists who, with far less expensive training, can do many of the same procedures (p. 161).

30. Studies have found that nurse-midwives provide care to significant numbers of poor and minority women. One 1992 study, in fact, found that 99 percent of certified nurse-midwives serve at least one group of vulnerable women, and that certified nurse-midwives (CNMs) in inner cities and rural areas serve several such groups. This study showed that few nurse-midwives practiced like obstetricians: only 11 percent of them were salaried, and 50 percent of their payments were from Medicaid and other government-sponsored programs; only 20 percent of their fees were of the traditional fee-for-service type. See Anne Scupholme et al., Jeanne DeJoseph, Donna M. Strobino, and Lisa L. Paine, "Nurse-midwifery Care to Vulnerable Populations. Phase 1: Demographic Characteristics of the National CNM Sample," *Journal of Nurse-Midwifery* 37 (1992): 341–348. A North Carolina program begun in the 1980s showed how one vulnerable population was being served by nurse-midwives. In 1988, the state instituted a program that offered to pay obstetricians' malpractice insurance if they agreed to practice in rural areas of the state that were drastically underserved. By 1991, the program was extended to cover certified nurse-midwives, whose mal-

practice costs were significantly lower. A 1992 study found that these nurse midwives maintained and even increased access to maternity care in these rural areas. See Donald H. Taylor et al., "One State's Response to the Malpractice Insurance Crisis: North Carolina's Rural Obstetrical Care Incentive Program," *Public Health Reports* 107 (1992): 523–529.

Appendix

1. For coding occupation for this and all of the succeeding data sets, I used the categories defined by the Federal Census of 1940: professional; managers and administrators; clerical and office workers; salesmen; farming, fishing and lumbering; mining and quarrying; transport and delivery; skilled craftsmen; nonskilled workers; service. The categories are roughly hierarchical, except for the two categories in the middle, farming and mining. To approximate white-collar and blue-collar occupations, I grouped the professional, managerial, clerical, and sales categories together as white collar, and the transport, artisan, laborer, and service categories together as blue collar.

2. To assess urban and rural differences in the pilot study, I divided Dane County into six regions. The city of Madison formed the first region, and succeeding regions formed concentric circles of increasing distance from Madison. For the data analysis used in the present study, I collapsed all of the rural regions outside of Madison into one region. Thus, place of birth collapsed into two categories: urban or rural.

3. I used fourteen categories for both mother's and father's place of birth: Dane County; Other Wisconsin; Other United States; Norway; Sweden and Denmark; Germany, Prussia, Bohemia, and Pomerania; England and Scotland; Ireland; Italy; Switzerland; Other North America; Other European; Other; and Unknown. Because the father's birthplace was noted more often than the mother's birthplace, for most analyses, I took the father's birthplace as representative of the entire family's ethnic identity.

4. Birth problems were not noted very often on the birth certificates, and it is difficult to know if they always were noted when they occurred. The categories I coded were the following: stillborn; forceps used; premature but baby lived; baby born alive but died short time after birth; long labor; mother died; another attendant assisted; none; unknown.

5. The attendant's home was coded in the same way as the parents' residence.

6. The categories for this variable were: physician; midwife; health officer; priest or minister; parents; and unknown.

7. Judith Walzer Leavitt studied the politics of health reform in Milwaukee in *The Healthiest City: Milwaukee and the Politics of Health Reform* (Princeton: Princeton University Press, 1982). Kathleen Neils Conzen assessed the early immigrant experience in *Immigrant Milwaukee, 1836–1860: Accommodation and Community in a Frontier City,* Harvard Studies in Urban History (Cambridge: Harvard University Press, 1976). Roger Simons' work on Milwaukee neighborhoods was also quite important; see "The City-Building Process: Housing and Services in New Milwaukee Neighborhoods, 1880–1910," *Transactions of the American Philosophical Society* 68, pt. 5 (1978).

8. Merle Eugene Curti, *The Making of an American Community; A Case Study of*

Democracy in a Frontier County, with the assistance of Robert Daniel et al. (Stanford: Stanford University Press, 1959).

9. Price County had developed as a prime logging area when the railroads moved north. After 1900, agriculture replaced logging, and the number of farms increased dramatically.

10. To avoid possible biases in reporting births in relation to the seasons, I tried to code months that spanned two seasons. Because winter births were often reported much later than those of other seasons, I did not code any of the winter months. Thus, for 1873 and 1877, I coded births from February, March, April, and May. In 1880, I coded births for April, May, June, and July. For the sampled years between 1885 and 1920, I coded the months of May, June, and July.

11. I coded the births for the months between January and June when I coded for six months in Trempealeau and Price Counties.

12. Place of birth was coded as: home, hospital, other.

13. The occupation categories were the same ones used for the Dane County data set. However, the category for farming, fishing, and lumbering was limited by the county. Thus, in Milwaukee County this category referred to fishing, and in Trempealeau or Price County it referred to farming or lumbering.

14. Mother's and father's birthplace were both coded with the following categories: Germany; Switzerland; Norway, Denmark, and Sweden; Greece; Austria-Hungary; Poland; Italy; Finland; Bohemia; Russia; Ireland; France; England; Canada; Europe (not specified or other); Wisconsin; United States (not Wisconsin). However, because the father's birthplace was listed more frequently, it was used in the analysis of ethnicity.

15. Parity was not always noted, but I coded for it when it did appear.

16. Categories for complications included: stillborn; forceps used; baby born alive, then died; twins; premature; doctor assisted midwife; illegitimate.

17. Categories coded included midwife, doctor, health officer, clergy, parent, other.

18. There were twenty-eight hospitals in Milwaukee and one hospital, run by a physician, in Trempealeau County.

19. I identified 893 midwives and 1,149 physicians in the four counties through birth certificates.

20. The Census Department administered the Birth Registration Area, which each state joined voluntarily. To join, however, each state had to have at least 90 percent of their births registered. A study of childbirth conditions in Marathon County during the second decade of the twentieth century revealed that of 110 unregistered births, 42 were known to be attended by physicians and 44 were known to be attended by midwives. Of the 44 unregistered midwife births, all but 15 were from one Polish settlement, where one midwife was not reporting the births she attended. The survey authors concluded that, on the whole, midwives had as good a record in their reporting of births as physicians. Florence Brown Sherbon and Elizabeth Moore, *Maternity and Infant Care in Two Rural Counties in Wisconsin,* U.S. Department of Labor, Children's Bureau Publication no. 46 (Washington, D.C.: Government Printing Office, 1919), p. 34.

21. Births attended by neighbor-woman midwives may be underrepresented. The State of Wisconsin Board of Health Report for 1914–15 noted, for example, that the greatest problem in reporting births was where there was no attendant. "With but few exceptions, the physicians and midwives are reporting their births very promptly,

but where the only attendant at the birth is some neighbor woman, unless the parents realize the importance of registering the birth, no record is made in a large number of cases." C. A. Harper, *Twenty-Sixth Report of the State Board of Health of Wisconsin for the Term Ending June 30th, 1916, with Report of the State Bureau of Vital Statistics for the Calendar Years of 1914 and 1915* (Madison: State Printer, 1917), p. 169.

22. Statutes of Wisconsin, Section 6933, paragraph 5. The number of births affected by this law, however, was small. The State of Wisconsin Board of Health Report for 1909, for example, showed 6 illegitimate births in Dane County, 6 in Trempealeau County, 2 in Price County, and 278 in Milwaukee. These births were 0.4 percent of births in Dane County, 0.1 percent in Trempealeau County, 0.7 percent in Price County, and 2.5 percent in Milwaukee County. C. A. Harper, *Twenty-Third Report of the State Board of Health of Wisconsin for the Two Years Ending September 30, 1910, together with the State Bureau of Vital Statistics for the Calendar Years of 1909 and 1910* (Madison: State Printer, 1912), p. 117, table 6.

23. Categories included: Milwaukee; Chicago; New York City; Minnesota; St. Louis; New York State; Illinois; Louisiana; Wisconsin; Germany; Austria; Bohemia; Hungary; Luxembourg; Norway; Russia; Sweden; Poland; Switzerland; Italy; and Rumania.

24. For this data set as well as the midwives' state licenses, I used a three-digit code. The first digit denoted country, the next two, the school. Thus, the schools could be collapsed by country. The school categories included: Germany, twenty-two schools; Switzerland and Italy, eight schools; Denmark, Norway, and Sweden, six schools; Greece, Yugoslavia, three schools; Austria-Hungary, including Bohemia, twenty-eight schools; Milwaukee, nine schools (included doctors who trained apprentices); Chicago and St. Louis, eleven schools; Poland and Russia, six schools; Great Britain, three schools; and United States, eleven schools.

25. Every physician giving a reference was given a number—there were forty-six different physicians.

26. See Wisconsin Statutes, Chapter 528, §1435f-12 (1909).

27. For a detailed description of the politics leading up to the passage of this bill, see Mary Elizabeth Fiorenza, "Midwifery and the Law in Illinois and Wisconsin, 1877–1917" (master's thesis, University of Wisconsin—Madison, 1985). The criteria are detailed on pp. 75–76.

28. Categories included married, divorced, single, and unknown.

29. Categories included college, apprentice, doctor, and none.

30. See description of colleges in n. 24.

31. The county where each doctor reference lived was noted.

32. Each doctor was assigned a number there were at least 238 different doctors.

33. For midwives from the four counties in the birth certificate study, each layperson was assigned a number; most were clergymen. There were 80 different names.

34. The survey by Florence Sherbon and Elizabeth Moore found that many midwives in the county had never applied for certificates of registration. However, most of these midwives only went out as a courtesy for their neighbors. Two midwives in Sherbon and Moore's survey, whom they considered "professionals," did have state licenses (Sherbon and Moore, *Maternity and Infant Care,* pp. 30–32).

35. Midwife categories included midwife, housewife, nurse, doctor, and other; Physician categories included doctor, pharmacist, and other. Only a very few physicians were not listed as such in the census.

36. Categories included: Germany (including Prussia); Switzerland; Italy; Norway, Denmark, or Sweden; Finland; Greece; Austria-Hungary; Bohemia; Poland; Russia; Ireland; England; France; Europe; Wisconsin; United States; and Canada.

37. The same categories were used for parents' birthplace as for the birth attendant's birthplace.

38. See categories for Dane County birth certificate study in n. 1.

39. Categories employed were nuclear, extended, boarders, and other.

40. Simon found that German and Polish families were tied for first place in 1900 in the percentage of private families owning homes. See Roger D. Simon, "The City-Building Process," p. 18.

41. "Directory of Milwaukee Physicians, 1834–1914: Years of Practice[;] School and Degree[;] Specialties," in Louis Frederick Frank, *The Medical History of Milwaukee, 1834–1914* (Milwaukee: Germania Publishing Co., 1915), pp. 238–271.

42. Wisconsin Statutes, Chapter 87, section 1.

43. The Physician's Register is numbered as Series 1621, Board of Medical Examiners, Register of Physicians. The thirty-three boxes of licenses that covered the period between 1899 and 1930 are part of Series 1606, Board of Medical Examiners, Applications for Licenses, Physicians.

44. I coded physicians' medical schools in the same manner as I coded midwife colleges. Each school was given a three-digit code, the first digit representing the state or country where the school was located. Thus, the many categories of medical colleges could be collapsed into a smaller number of categories that incorporated the countries where these schools were located. The school categories were as follows: Norway, two schools; Austria, two schools; Wisconsin, five schools; Germany, twelve schools; Poland, one school; England, Scotland, and Canada, four schools; and United States, seventy schools.

45. Schools of practice included regular, homeopathic, eclectic, osteopathic, and physiomedical.

46. The specialist categories included none, surgery, obstetrics, oncology, rectal diseases, and insanity. Though few doctors in this time period were specialists, the language of the license form probably discouraged most doctors from reporting any specialty. The line on the license form asked if the doctor "practised as an Advertising Specialist, or Itinerant Physician, or do you contemplate doing so?"

47. The categories used here were the same ones used for the birth certificates and for the census study.

48. Appeared as a line after 1912. However, this variable was not consistently reported. See the discussion in chapter 5.

49. See John Beffel, "Comments," for Dorothy Reed Mendenhall, "Prenatal and Natal Conditions in Wisconsin," *Wisconsin Medical Journal* 15 (1917): 366.

50. See Marija J. Norusis, *SPSS/PC+: For the IBM PC/XT/AT* (Chicago: SPSS, 1986); also Norusis, *SPSS/PC+: Advanced Statistics for the IBM PC/XT/AT* (Chicago: SPSS, 1986).

51. Morris Hamburg, *Basic Statistics: A Modern Approach,* 3rd ed. (San Diego: Harcourt Brace Jovanovich, 1985), pp. 128–131.

Index

abortion, 154–155, 242n9
African-American midwives, 2, 4, 15, 18, 19, 157, 245n21
Alabama, midwives in, 18, 19, 157
American Association of Obstetricians and Gynecologists, 115, 136
American Board of Obstetrics and Gynecology, 115, 149–150
American College of Obstetricians and Gynecologists, 150, 158
American Gynecological Society, 33, 115
American Medical Association, 114–115, 131, 146
American Medical Association, Council on Medical Education, 92, 103
American Midwife, The, 25
apprentice training: midwives, 13, 15, 17–21, 35, 58, 86; physicians, 28, 94, 99, 101
Arms, Suzanne, 158
Augusta, Maine, 66–67
Austro-Hungarian midwives, 25
automobiles, in physician practice, 125, 136, 232n19

Ballard, Martha, 10, 66–67, 183n7, 243n12
Bellevue Hospital School for Midwives (New York City), 26, 33, 34, 187n58
Boston, midwives in, 52, 74

Carnegie Foundation, 101
"catching babies," defined, 179n16
cesarean sections, 148, 234n24
Chicago, midwives in, 52, 242n9
Children's Bureau, 16, 19, 44, 54, 57, 60–61, 64, 113, 198n10, 221–222n12
Cleveland, physicians in, 118
Conzen, Kathleen, 10

country doctors. *See* general practitioners; rural physicians.
Curti, Merle, 180n24

Dane County: midwives in, 41, 45, 55, 56, 57–59, 65–67; physicians in, 124–125, 145, 230n6
Davis, Michael, 43
DeLee, Joseph B., 7, 100, 109, 131, 156, 157; on midwives, 43–44
Deutiche Hebammen Schule (Chicago), 26–27
Dick-Read, Grantly, 158
direct-entry midwives, 204n12
druggists and physicians, 122, 225n39

education, medical, 6, 13, 14, 90–116, 142, 229n72; before 1905, 93–101; cost of, 38–39; post-1905, 101–116
education, midwife, 13–36, 55, 57, 77; in Europe, 24–25
education, nursing, 13, 14
Eliot, Charles, 94
Engelmann, George J., 33, 97

Farmers' Institutes, 114
female physicians, 93, 152, 156, 158, 178n10, 180n23, 191n6, 233–234n23, 241–242n2, 246n28; social characteristics, 38–39
Finnish-American midwives, 45, 65, 153
Flexner, Abraham, 101, 103, 106, 110
Fraduate Midwifery School, Bergen, Norway, 54
France, midwives in, 186n49
Frank, Louis F., 92

Gaskin, Ina May, 158
gender theory, 192n15